"Morning sickness. Exhaust... parts of pregnancy are our greatest oppo... glory? In her beautiful book, Expectant, Heather Cofer reminds us that pregnancy is meant to be a nine month opportunity for worship. Share this book with every momma you know!"

Erin Davis
Author, blogger, podcaster, and momma of four.

"*Expectant* is a one-of-a-kind book about embracing all the stages of pregnancy from a gospel-centered perspective. What a gift for mothers-to-be and those who desire motherhood! We believe in the message of this book and hope it makes it into the hands of many expectant mothers."

Kristen Clark & Bethany Beal
Founders, GirlDefined Ministries
Authors of *Sex, Purity, and the Longings of a Girl's Heart*

"*Expectant* is a desperately needed gospel resource for pregnant women. As a first-time pregnant mom, I found this book to be a boon of encouragement, wisdom, grace, conviction, and joy. Reading it in my third trimester was an incredible blessing, and I'm so thankful for Heather Cofer and *Expectant.*"

Jaquelle Ferris
Author of *This Changes Everything*

"Pregnancy is sanctifying. Every step of the way, God is doing a work in our hearts to make us more like Jesus and more dependent on Him! In *Expectant*, Heather gives mamas hopeful reminders to look to Jesus throughout each trimester and in birth. Writing from her own experience, Heather offers practical tips and encouragement to help women walk through pregnancy with the joy of Christ during those nine months of grace upon grace."

Gretchen Saffles
Founder, Well-Watered Women

"Heather is the gentle and honest friend every pregnant woman needs. Heather's biblical guidance and personal stories point the fearful, anxious, and tired mom to the sufficiency of Christ. Pregnant moms who long to honor God will walk away from this book feeling refreshed and equipped to face pregnancy with joy and hope."

Lauren Washer
Writer

"In a world filled with lies about pregnancy and motherhood, Heather Cofer kindly and confidently points us back to the truth of Jesus. This book will help free you from the chains of socially acceptable self-focus and provide a vision for how beautiful a Christ-centered pregnancy can be for God's expectant daughters."

Naomi Vacaro
Founder, Wholehearted Quiet Time

"Heather writes with an honesty that helps the reader to see herself in the pages. Her commitment to the gospel is convicting and beautiful."

Jessica Mathisen
Author of *Choosing Contentment* and *Embracing Gratitude*

"Heather's book is written with such authenticity and realness, and yet, instead of using that as allowance to settle for mediocrity, is a desire to rise above, to rest in the arms of the One who is the Strength and Comfort during the both beautiful and challenging season of pregnancy. Being through five pregnancies myself, I know that her words are not just naive idealism; but rather a beautiful call to join hands together, a gentle beckoning to rise from self-absorption, and instead, to look to Jesus always."

Clarita Yoder
Blogger

Expectant

Cultivating a Vision for Christ-Centered Pregnancy

HEATHER COFER

Is. 26: 3-4

Heather Cofer

BURNING ❤ HEART

WINDSOR, COLORADO

Expectant

Edited by David Webb
Cover Design: Annie Wesche
Interior and Digital Design: Michael Morgan

First Printing 2020

Paperback ISBN: 978-1-952513-01-5
Mobipocket ISBN: 978-1-952513-00-8

This book is dedicated to my husband, Judah, for constantly cheering me on and leading me well.

And to our moms, who are the ultimate examples of the words in this book.

Contents

ACKNOWLEDGMENTS

My deepest thanks goes to every one of you who have supported me in so many ways throughout this process. To my parents, for the years of investing in my life and cheering me on. To my siblings and dear friends who provided insight and encouragement when I needed it most. Thank you Ella, Elsje, Carol Beth (Mom), Brooke, Shelly, Lauren, Trina (Mom Cofer), Emily, and Michelle for sharing your testimonies and for allowing the Lord to grow you and use you during your pregnancies. I've been incredibly blessed and directed to Jesus by each of your lives.

Thank you, Ervina, for being willing to share your story of looking to Jesus in the face of incredible loss. Thank you for allowing it to encourage others who are walking a similar path. I am so grateful for your heart and have found a kindred spirit in you.

Thank you, Jasmin, for being my faithful editor and cheerleader during this whole process, and for sharing your own story of God's faithfulness on your journey of infertility. I am beyond thankful that God has gifted me with your friendship.

Thank you, Leslie, for the many years you have invested into my life as part of the Set Apart Girl team and for being a mentor in my writing journey. It has been such an honor and privilege to work alongside you to encourage women in their walk with the Lord.

Thank you, Ann, for the time you invested and the insight you've shared from your years of publishing experience. It's been invaluable and an encouragement many times over.

Thank you, Annie, for the beautiful cover design and promotional graphics, for your encouragement over the years, and for your example of trusting Jesus in all things.

Thank you to my incredible editor, David, for taking my words and making them better than I could have ever made them on my own.

Thank you, Michael, for helping bring the book to fruition with your formatting skills.

Thank you, Cristina, for being an amazing proofreader and all-round encouragement.

Thank you to my kiddos, who have been used mightily by the Lord to grow me from the moment they were conceived. Each of you is a precious gift.

Thank you, my beloved Judah, for being such a faithful leader in this endeavor (and for giving me the idea in the first place). Thank you for providing strength, encouragement, comfort, and truth during each pregnancy, and at every stage of writing this book. I could not have done it without you, and I thank God continually that He has given me such an incredible husband and father for our children.

And thank you most of all to Jesus Christ, my Savior and King. Without you, I would have no hope. Apart from you, there would have been no book to write. I am eternally grateful that you have given me new life and enabled me by your Spirit to live in obedience to you. May you receive all the glory!

FOREWORD

My husband, Eric, and I were married for ten years before we had children. The official reason for this rather long delay—i.e., the answer we gave to anyone nosy enough to ask—was that we were incredibly busy with ministry and travel and were waiting to start a family until our lives settled down a bit.

But in all honesty, there was a deeper reason for my reluctance to say yes to the pitter-patter of little feet: After talking with a number of women who described motherhood as a chaotic and exhausting experience, I had become afraid of having children. Pregnancy was another reason for my hesitation. I dreaded the idea of enduring morning sickness, gaining weight, and losing sleep, not to mention the labor-and-delivery process itself. Growing up, I'd always desired to be a mom someday. But as a woman, I had become convinced that pregnancy and motherhood would take a tremendous toll on my life, and I didn't feel ready for it.

After years of struggle, I asked God to change my heart toward having children. As I searched the Scriptures in the wake of this prayer, I was excited to discover that the Lord's purpose for motherhood is to bring *strength* into our lives, not weakness. (See Psalm 127 and 113:9, for example.) But I also learned that in God's plan, the key to finding strength and joy in motherhood comes from approaching it with an entirely different attitude—one that no longer asks, "What can I get?" but rather, "What can I *give*?"

Embracing this shift of perspective was a turning point in my life. By God's grace, I said yes to the inconveniences and sacrifices of pregnancy and motherhood, and I have never regretted it for a moment.

That's why I'm thrilled that Heather Cofer has written this book. *Expectant* shows us that motherhood, from the moment of conception on, provides an amazing opportunity for us to deny ourselves, embrace sacrificial love, and follow in the footsteps of our Lord Jesus Christ. Heather does a beautiful job of weaving together biblical principles and candid personal stories to capture a vision for pregnancy that goes far beyond baby showers and maternity clothes. This book inspires us to view pregnancy through God's eyes and shows us how this "expectant season" can draw us closer to the Source of all life.

Having worked with Heather for many years through our magazine, *Set Apart Girl*, and observing her life through pregnancy and motherhood, I can attest that this book is an outflow of what she has lived. Though *Expectant* presents a counterculture message, it is delivered with grace, love, and heartfelt honesty that is both refreshing and encouraging.

As you read this book, I encourage you to let the Lord personally speak to your heart and gently refine your approach to pregnancy and motherhood, whether you are expecting your first child or your tenth. When you willingly embrace this season as an opportunity to glorify God, you'll discover the amazing joy that comes through offering your body as a living sacrifice to the One who gave everything for you. Truly, He is worthy.

Leslie Ludy

Bestselling author of *The Set Apart Woman* and
Set Apart Motherhood

Introduction

EXPECTING A MIRACLE

*For by him all things were created, in heaven and on earth
... all things were created through him and for him. And
he is before all things, and in him all things hold together.*
Colossians 1:16–17

In his pioneering work *An American Dictionary of the English Language,* devout Christian and prolific author Noah Webster defined the word *expectant* as an adjective meaning "waiting" or "looking for." As a noun, *expectant* was defined by Webster as "one who waits in expectation" or "one held in dependence by his belief or hope of receiving some good."[1]

Expectant is a beautiful word that describes both the mom-to-be *and* the family's happy anticipation of welcoming a new life into the home. But as Webster knew, it also paints a vivid picture of the fruitful Christian life. The true believer is a faithful steward of the Lord's household, one who chooses each day to put others first, to love and serve Christ's family with joy while also preparing and watching for His return. The true believer walks by faith daily, held in dependence on God's provision by the belief and hope that He rewards those who diligently seek Him (Hebrews 11:6).

It's this eager expectation I hope to communicate to you through this book: that as you seek to keep Jesus Christ at the center of your family and your pregnancy, He will work His power in and through you to bring new life into your home and your community.

It's All About Jesus

God was walking me through an incredible journey even before I conceived my first child. He had already begun stirring in my heart the desire for something more than what is considered "normal" in pregnancy and to walk through it in a way that brings Him great glory by displaying to all I come into contact with that God is the giver of life and the provider of everything a mom needs to carry a new little life with joy, peace, and grace in every circumstance.

What He has shown me in countless ways on this journey is that pregnancy, contrary to what the world will say, is *not* ultimately about the mom or even the baby. It is about Jesus, just as every sphere and season of a life ought to be. Pregnancy, with all its unique challenges and joys, is simply another way to allow the Lord to work in our lives, to draw us closer to Him while also pointing others to His infinite love.

Pregnancy is a time for the mom-to-be to prepare to raise the child growing in her womb in the fear and admonition of the Lord. It is a time for her to prepare to serve and love that little person unconditionally. It is a time for her to grow in mental and emotional strength while yet deepening her dependence on the Lord to help her fulfill well her calling as a mother.

My own journey through four pregnancies (so far) has brought some of the deepest joys of my life, but it has also presented some of the most difficult emotional and physical trials I've ever experienced. Yet in each of these mountains and valleys, I have seen God's goodness and faithfulness displayed over and over again as I held fast to Him and allowed Him to grow me through the journey.

As I have labored (no pun intended) for several years now to put these words on paper, my desire has always been this: that each of you who reads this will catch a vision for honoring Christ in the season of pregnancy and be greatly encouraged that, as His child, you have been given all you need to do so. Whether you are in the midst of pregnancy, have yet to become pregnant, or have walked through several already, I pray that this book will be a great encouragement and inspire you to grow ever more in love with Jesus Christ.

Laborers of Love

I have been so blessed to be surrounded by women who have also walked through pregnancy with a desire to honor the Lord. I have asked a few of them to share part of their stories at the end of each chapter so that you can catch a glimpse into how they intentionally dedicated themselves and their little ones to Him. Some of these women have had one or two children, while others have had eight, but all of them can beautifully testify to God's goodness and faithfulness. A few are very dear friends and peers of mine, while others are precious mentors in my life. I know you will be challenged and encouraged by each of them, just as I have been.

At the end of the book, you will find a pair of "bonus" chapters on topics I have very little or no experience in, but which I felt were important to address when talking about pregnancy. For each of these chapters, I asked a mom who has been an incredible example in this area to write in my stead. If you have walked through loss or infertility, I pray that you will be greatly blessed and heartened by their words. In any case, I pray that you will find in these chapters a greater understanding and willingness to love and support the ones who have traversed these roads.

Finally, I pray that through this book you will be filled with hope and expectation in seeing the beauty that a Christ-centered pregnancy can hold.

1

My Story

*"For as the heavens are higher than the earth, so are my ways
higher than your ways and my thoughts than your thoughts."*
Isaiah 55:9

On a warm September afternoon, I found myself driving to
the grocery store for the purpose of buying a single item: a
pregnancy test. *Settle down,* I said to myself. *You're not taking
a test because you think you're pregnant. You're just ruling it out
so you can tell the doctor you're definitely not pregnant. Don't get
your hopes up again.*

Time after time I had purchased that two-pack of little white
sticks, dutifully followed the instructions, and waited, longing for
that second line to appear. And every time my hope would turn
to grief as I stared at yet another negative. This time, though, I
was determined not to be disappointed, because I was certain I
wasn't pregnant. I had experienced some recent health problems,
and I just needed to be able to tell my doctor at an upcoming
appointment that they weren't the result of pregnancy. That's
why I hadn't said anything about it to my husband. I didn't want
him to be disappointed again either.

This time, as I waited for the results, I was reluctant to look. But I watched in utter shock as that faint second line appeared and darkened into the positive I had wondered if I'd ever see.

From the time I was about five, my dream was to grow up, get married, and have children. I am the second of eight children. I was the oldest girl, so that may have contributed to my love of little ones. I would gaze at a newborn baby in church, hoping the mom would see the longing in my eyes and let me snuggle her little one. I also couldn't wait to be pregnant! I remember being eleven or twelve and being so excited for the day when I could walk around with a baby bump. As I grew, my desire only increased, for I saw childbirth as a gift from the Lord.

As I neared the end of high school and began looking at various colleges and other educational opportunities I might pursue, a door never opened wide for me to step through and move forward. At the same time, my vision of being a wife and mother continued to grow and became more and more beautiful to me. It wasn't long after this that the Lord brought my husband into my life, confirming that this was where the Lord was leading me.

After getting married at the ripe old age of nineteen, I really had no desire to wait for children. But my husband, Judah, wasn't sure we should jump right into parenting so soon. The Lord took us through a process of praying and giving that area of our lives to Him, and I was *so* excited when, six months later, Judah said he felt good about starting to actively try for a child.

Of course, I kind of expected I would become pregnant right away. My mom had never had any problem getting pregnant, so I assumed it would be the same for me. But after a few months of trying, nothing had happened. I had been diligent about tracking my cycles and was confused as to why this "wasn't working." I had been experiencing some strange health issues for several years prior to getting married, so I decided to have them checked out, thinking there might be a connection.

Letting Go

A few days after visiting the doctor and undergoing some tests, he called with a diagnosis that will be forever etched in my mind: "From the results of the ultrasound, it looks like you have Polycystic Ovarian Syndrome." I had no idea what it was, so as soon as I got off the phone with him, I got on my computer and looked it up.

I was absolutely devastated.

One symptom for this condition stood out like a neon sign: "infertility." No, I thought, I have always wanted this! This has been my dream. I want children so badly. This can't be real!

That summer was one of the toughest periods of my life as I grappled with the reality that I might never have biological children. Only a few close friends and family knew what we were facing. So when we began getting well-meaning hints from friends about starting a family, we would just smile and say we were trusting the Lord's timing. But every well-meaning comment felt like salt in a wound.

I was trying to walk a tightrope of being willing to accept the possibility I would never get pregnant while still remaining hopeful. But in those months, I felt the Lord asking me to give that up. He gently showed me that having children was something I had made an idol in my life—something I longed for more than Him. I felt Him saying to me, *Do you trust that I am enough? Even if you never have children of your own, do you believe that you have everything you need to be completely fulfilled and joyful in Me?*

After a summer filled with tears and much painful wrestling, I surrendered my desire for children to the Lord. Even though I *felt* that having biological kids would be the best thing for me,

I knew I ultimately wanted *His* best for me. Most days I had to remind myself of this truth and lay my desire again at His feet whenever I felt those pangs of longing for my womb to be filled. Through that process, I began to see Christ's peace and joy manifesting itself in my life in a much deeper way. The pain was still strong at times, but I knew where to take it.

One Sunday near the end of September, our pastor preached a sermon on raising children to be world changers for the sake of the gospel. Both Judah and I were so moved by the sermon, and that night we prayed together and asked the Lord to prepare us for whatever children would look like for us—biological, adopted, or spiritual—and help us to disciple them to love and serve Jesus with their whole lives. It was then that it struck me, *really* struck me, that having children goes far beyond simply raising and enjoying and loving little people; it is an intentional, deeply significant process of pointing young ones to Jesus and training them to give themselves fully to Him. Although I still had no idea if or when I would ever have my own children, I had gained a vision for something very precious.

Surprised by Joy

One week later, we graduated from Ellerslie Discipleship Training, which we had been attending for a year. This had been a beautiful season of spiritual growth for both Judah and me and had greatly impacted the foundations of both our lives and our marriage. At this point we weren't exactly sure what our next steps would be, but we were excited for whatever the Lord had for us.

This brings me back to that September afternoon as I stared at my first positive pregnancy test. Shaking and wide-eyed, I remember the whispered words "No way . . . no way" falling from my mouth. When I went to the office and tried to tell Judah, all I could say was, "Um . . . uh . . . I, uh. . . ." His eyes got really big. He could tell from the look on my face that something really significant was happening. As he started walking toward me, he asked, "Are you pregnant?" All I could do was nod in response. We were so overwhelmed by God's gift to us! Right then and there, we prayed for the little life that was forming inside of me, thanking the Lord for entrusting us with this child.[1]

I certainly wouldn't have chosen that path to childbirth, with its difficulties, the weeping, and the heartbreak of facing the possibility of infertility. But I am so thankful for the way the Lord used those things to reshape my mindset from "I deserve this" to being able to humbly—and with a heart overflowing with thanksgiving—accept this as a precious gift I wasn't worthy of.

Judah asked me, after the reality began to sink in, "Well, what should we do to get ready?" I laughed and said, "I guess right now we just … wait." (We decided prayer and reading parenting books should be added to the list, too). Little did I know the how the Lord was going to use those months of waiting to shape me, humble me, and grow me, not only in preparation for motherhood but also to sanctify every area of my life.

During this season of growth, God began laying on my heart a vision of something more for the nine months of pregnancy—something different from what this world would say is "normal." I found I wanted to glorify Him in every moment, not just after the morning sickness (read: all-day sickness) had passed or when my emotions were stable. I longed to overcome the frequent temptation to give in to self-indulgence, laziness, irritability, grumpiness, or fear. Instead, I was determined to find my joy in Christ even in the most difficult moments. After having just walked through the dark days of thinking I might not be able to bear children, I wanted to be just as committed to glorifying the Lord in pregnancy as I had been in surrendering this area of my life to Him and letting go of my dreams.

As I sought the Lord daily and committed my pregnancy to Him, He did amazing work in my life. There were many times

I cried out to Him, keenly aware of my deep need for Jesus and His strength. And every time I did, He abundantly answered. He showed me His faithfulness over and over again, and that first pregnancy became one of the most beautiful chapters in my life. I'm excited to share more about this time in the pages to come.

Faithful Again

Shortly after the first birthday of our son, Jude, I learned I was pregnant again. I was elated at this precious new life growing inside of me. But when, at five weeks, I woke up feeling the full force of morning sickness (triggered by the smell of coffee, one of my favorite things), I was reminded that this wasn't going to be a walk in the park. I had to be just as diligent in seeking the Lord as I had been the first time around, and this time I had a rambunctious toddler to care for.

Yet I knew that the grace He had given the first time would be just as readily available to me. And again I experienced the amazing, enabling grace of God in beautiful, inexpressible ways. Through all of my foibles and failures in attitudes, actions, and words, He was faithful to grow me, sanctify me, and draw me closer to Him.

During this pregnancy, through some unexpected circumstances, I was pushed to a greater level of selflessness and servant-heartedness than I had ever experienced. At the very time I had planned to work on this book, God was qualifying me to write the things He had placed on my heart through having me walk them out moment by moment. He showed me in very real ways that His grace was sufficient all the time, in every situation, and that there was never a second I needed to give in to selfishness or fear. Rather, I could live in an abundance of joy and peace and a continual outpouring of love for those around me.

Yes, there were times when every bone in my body wanted to give in to self-pity and indulgence of the flesh under the justification of being pregnant. But whenever I gave in to those feelings, I always regretted it. When I instead turned my eyes upon Jesus, there was always the strength I needed to live for Him and be His hands and feet to the people around me.

And the Third Time ... and a Fourth

In December 2016, we welcomed our third child, Jeneva, into the world. Just when I was beginning to think that I had learned everything I could from pregnancy, this time I faced a whole new set of challenges, from deep emotional struggles to the possibility of complications with our daughter shortly before her birth.

During labor, we faced the possibility of an emergency C-section and saw the power of prayer to turn the situations into a testimony of His power. I was forced to cling to Jesus more fiercely than ever before, and I could see more clearly than ever that He was my only hope. And all the while, many of the same things He had taught me during my first two pregnancies were more deeply imbedded in my soul.

Last year, we had our fourth child, Javan. That pregnancy came with its own unexpected physical difficulties, and I needed another dose of resolve to keep my eyes fixed upon Jesus and "rejoice always" (1 Thessalonians 5:16), which seemed to be the theme of that pregnancy. As I reread the chapters of this manuscript, it served as fresh encouragement, motivation, and conviction that the Lord had yet again given me all I needed to walk through pregnancy in a way that glorifies Him in every facet of the journey.

Catching a Vision for Pregnancy

Pregnancy is such a unique season of life. It is a time of great sweetness and joy, coupled with the expectancy and anticipation of what is to come. There are also all the challenges of handling hormonal changes, coping with morning sickness, and facing the fear of the what-ifs. But God's desire for every woman walking through pregnancy, whether it goes as smoothly as can be or is filled with trials, is that this time be glorifying to Him. He desires that every season of life—whether joyful or difficult, peaceful or filled with suffering—be a testimony of His life within us. The apostle Paul writes in Colossians 3:17, "Whatever you do, in word or in deed, do everything in the name of the Lord Jesus." He doesn't say "except when you're pregnant—then you can do and say whatever you like." If we are indeed new creations in Christ (2 Corinthians 5:17), then every season of life is a new opportunity to walk according to the power of the Holy Spirit who dwells in us.

Don't get me wrong. I'm the first to admit that pregnancy is hard. It does not always feel wonderful and glow-y like we imagine it to be before experiencing it ourselves. But the Lord often uses the difficult seasons of our lives to grow us most. And these times are also when others can see there truly is a difference between those who believe in Jesus and those who do not. When we are filled with joy, hope, and peace in the midst of life's toughest trials, Jesus will shine brightly through us to those with whom we interact.

People have suggested that I've enjoyed easier-than-average pregnancies because I am young, and I don't deny that being young and healthy definitely helps. Nevertheless, I've still experienced debilitating bouts of morning sickness, severe nerve and back pain, sleepless nights, weeks of "false labor," the possibility of an unhealthy baby, and letting go of the desire for a natural birth. In each of these situations—and others like them—I had a choice to make. Would I give in to my flesh and wallow in self-pity and fear, or would I love and honor Jesus through each new obstacle? Would I rely on my own strength to get me through or choose to trust in God's enabling grace?

When God calls us to do something, He surely gives us all we need to carry it out. As the oft-quoted verse goes, "I can do all things through him who strengthens me" (Philippians 4:13). Pregnancy is no exception! Allow the Lord to give you His vision for what He desires to do in and through you during this time of carrying a new life.

As you read this book, I pray that you will be encouraged and challenged to see this season of life as a unique opportunity to experience and share the goodness, peace, strength, and joy of the Lord, through good days and hard days, from the moment you see that positive test to the day you hold that baby in your arms.

2

PREGNANCY AND WORSHIP

Draw near to God, and he will draw near to you.
James 4:8

I opened my eyes and looked at the clock. *It can't be 8:00 already!*
I'm still so tired, I thought as I tried to pull myself out of bed.
Nausea and exhaustion tried their hardest to draw me back under
the warm blankets, but I knew I needed to gather my wits and
get ready for the day.

A spoonful of peanut butter in hand, I sat down at the
dining room table to read my Bible. My head was still groggy,
and I struggled to grasp the concepts as I read and reread the
same passage. I was tempted to just set it aside this morning,
wondering if it was worth the effort. *Pregnancy brain is a real*
thing, I reasoned. *Too real.* But I kept going, trusting that my
sincere desire to seek the Lord and hide His word in my heart
would reap the fruit of righteousness (Philippians 1:11).

We had found out we were expecting our first child the day
after graduating from our year-long discipleship training program.
It had been an intense year of study and prayer, waking early and
spending many hours in God's presence. Before graduating, I

remember often thinking, *I am going to stay disciplined once we graduate. I'm going to keep the same schedule of Bible reading and prayer. I* will not *lose all the spiritual ground I've gained!* Well, as it turned out, it wasn't long before I could hardly drag myself out of bed in the mornings due to morning sickness and extreme fatigue and weakness (which I later found out was due partially to a major iron deficiency).

I quickly grew discouraged because I had wanted so badly to remain disciplined in spending time in the Word and prayer on a daily basis. Now it was all I could do at times to read one chapter or spend a few minutes in prayer.

One day, as I was sitting at the table, feeling defeated and very unspiritual, the Lord gently began challenging me. I remember "hearing" so clearly in my heart, *Why do you want to be disciplined? Is it simply for the sake of feeling good about yourself? Or is your desire truly to know Me more?*

I was so struck by this that my whole perspective began to change in that instant. I started to see that all the discipline in the world really means nothing if it is not for the sake of knowing and loving Jesus. Rather than becoming a mere task we tick off our checklist to feel more righteous, what He wants is a relationship with us.

I realized that God was not impressed with my study methods or commitment to a schedule. What He desired was for me to seek Him *every* moment of *every* day, walking in step with His Spirit (Galatians 5:25). He wanted me to come to Him with *every* joy and *every* difficulty and trust that He understands this season of life. (He designed it, after all.) I was always to be looking for the ways He wanted to use this season and its unique circumstances to teach me more about Himself.

Pregnancy Is a Poor Excuse

During my second pregnancy, my struggle was a bit different. Rather than being hard on myself for not spending every minute in the Word, I tended to excuse myself for not putting much effort toward it. My son was fifteen months old during the most difficult phase of my morning sickness. Jude was always active and wanted to explore everything, and it was all I could do to keep him from getting into trouble on his little adventures. When I put him down for his morning nap, I would often collapse onto the couch in a fatigued, nauseated heap. My first instinct was always to pick up my phone and begin browsing Instagram or Facebook. I would think, *God understands that I'm just too tired (or sick or foggy) to read Scripture today. I get so little quiet time. It's okay to spend it on something more mindless than praying or reading the Bible.*

Then I began to feel the prompting of God's Spirit: *If you have enough energy for social media, don't you think you have enough energy to spend time with Me? Do you not believe that true rest of mind and heart comes from being in My presence and delighting in Me?*

Without realizing it, I had gradually begun using the excuse "God understands" to justify spiritual laziness. As a result, my temper was shorter, my emotions were more volatile, and a mounting lack of self-control was evident in other areas of my life. I knew full well that if I had the mental capacity to navigate the internet, I certainly could use that time to cultivate my relationship with the Lord.

God was gracious to remind me that if I wanted to walk through pregnancy while pointing to Him with every aspect of my life, I had to completely depend upon Him. I couldn't pretend for one second that I was able to face the challenging moments in my own strength. (When I tried, I utterly failed anyway!) Just as He says, "Apart from me you can do nothing" (John 15:5).

Being Led by the Shepherd

One verse that was particularly comforting to me during pregnancy was Isaiah 40:11: "He will tend his flock like a shepherd; he will gather the lambs in his arms; he will carry them in his bosom, and gently lead those that are with young." God knows that pregnancy is often a very trying time in a woman's life; He doesn't beat us over the head when we're not able to maintain the same habits or schedule we had previously. The Lord is patient and gentle as we learn to traverse this new territory. And as the verse says, He gently *leads*. He is right there with us, never leaving or forsaking us. When we start to veer off course, He gives us a gentle tap with His rod and brings us back to His path.

Submitting to His leading is the key to walking out a Christ-centered pregnancy. We absolutely *cannot* rely on our own resolve. Hormones are raging and emotions are volatile. The physical changes alone can cause us to feel more insecure, while all the unknowns linger in the back of the mind, making us more susceptible to irrationality and fear. Pregnancy is the perfect time to see that His grace is sufficient and His power made perfect in our weakness (2 Corinthians 12:9).

Choosing His Grace

Near the beginning of my first pregnancy, someone said something that hurt my feelings terribly. I knew this person was completely oblivious to my pain, but I allowed my emotions to take control. After days of wrestling with this, I finally sobbed the story to my husband. "I have tried to forgive [this person], but I feel like it's impossible," I said through my tears.

I will never forget Judah's next words: "But Heather, you *have* to. You cannot hold this against them. Just ask Jesus for His help, and ask Him to bless them."

So although my emotions were telling me I was still angry and had a right to be bitter, I chose to obey the Lord. There, on the edge of our bed with my husband's arm around me, I choked out a prayer, forgiving this person and asking the Lord to bless them. And once I did, all the bitterness melted away. My obedience had reaped faith and freedom from the bondage of unforgiveness.

Pregnant or otherwise, we will never face a situation in which God will not give us what we need to walk in obedience to Him. Yes, sometimes joy truly does feel out of reach when we're nauseated day and night and our emotions make no sense. It is in those moments we must choose to walk by faith, not by feelings. We have to turn to God's Word and remember His promises:

> *Let us then with confidence draw near to the throne of grace, that we may receive mercy and find grace to help in time of need. (Hebrews 4:16)*

> *I know how to be brought low, and I know how to abound. In any and every circumstance, I have learned the secret of facing plenty and hunger, abundance and need. I can do all things through him who strengthens me. (Philippians 4:12–13)*

Paul, who we know wrote at least one of these verses, experienced many, many difficulties in his life and ministry. I'm sure being whipped and stoned are just as hard, if not more so, than many of the things a woman deals with during pregnancy. Yet Paul was able to rejoice and be content. What was his secret? Jesus. He was fully dependent on the life of Jesus in him, and he trusted that God's grace would enable him to endure each and every trial.

It's so wonderful to know that the same Holy Spirit who lived in Paul also dwells in each of us who are God's children! We have access to all the joy, all the peace, and all the hope that has been available to each and every follower of Christ who has ever lived. All we need do is believe what God says and act upon it.

The strength to do this comes by seeking God daily, even moment by moment. When we continually delight in Him and enjoy His presence, when we long with all our hearts to know and love Him, He will unfailingly fill us with joy, peace, patience, and every other fruit of His Spirit. And each time we choose to act by faith rather than our feelings, we will see God's promises fulfilled in our lives and our faith will grow.

It Takes Intentionality

I've learned that if I want to accomplish a goal I've set for myself, it hardly ever just "happens." If I have the urge to do a deep clean of the kitchen or prepare a fancy dinner, I can't simply depend on moments of free time magically opening up during my day. No, I have to intentionally plan my day and each of the events in it to accommodate doing that particular thing.

The same concept applies to time alone with the Lord. If I am not intentional about planning my day so that I can have time with the Lord, it very easily gets pushed aside by the many other things demanding my attention. And if I'm not diligent to seek the Lord during seasons of pregnancy, I soon find myself at the mercy of my emotions.

On the days I wake up saying, "Lord, I want to glorify you today—help me to recognize each moment how I can display your life in me, and enable me to do pregnancy better than I can in my own strength," I find I am continually aware of ways in which I can grow spiritually and glorify the Lord through my actions and reactions. On these days, I more readily choose to deny selfishness and laziness, and I repent of sin quickly. And during these days I see a marked difference for the better in my attitude and perspective.

This is the foundation of a Christ-centered pregnancy. I can try to muster up the willpower to plaster on a smile when I don't feel good, be super self-disciplined in my diet and exercise, or even maintain our home and craft a flawless birth plan. But if I try to accomplish these things in my own strength, I'm bound to run out at some point. These things must flow out of my love for Jesus and be done in the strength *He* provides.

I don't know if you are struggling with one extreme or the other—either beating yourself up about not being disciplined or making excuses to give into laziness (maybe some of both)—but here are a few different strategies that can be helpful in building a strong relationship with the Lord during the season of pregnancy.

Listen to the Bible

While I was pregnant with my son Jude, I began listening to an audio recording of the Bible. I found this to be a wonderful way to saturate my mind and heart with truth throughout the day. I continued to do this after Jude was born, and now he too has listened to the whole Bible through several times.

Sometimes when it is hard for me to focus my eyes to read, I will just lie down and listen to Scripture or play it while driving or getting ready in the morning. Listening to the Word while folding laundry or doing dishes is very helpful in keeping my focus on the Lord all day long.

Keep a Prayer Journal

I've had terrible brain fog with all my pregnancies, and so I often struggled to maintain focus while praying. I have found that keeping a prayer journal helps me to be more intentional and mindful during my prayer times. Once I spend a little time writing, I find that I'm able to set aside my journal and just talk with the Lord. This habit sets a precedent for the rest of my day as well.

Keeping a journal can help you home in on two or three specific things to pray for. It's also a great way to record praise reports and answered prayers. Journal with *much* thanksgiving, and in those inevitable hard moments, you'll be able to look back on to all the things you have to be thankful for: His salvation, His love, His protection, His patience, His faithfulness—the list goes on and on!

Seek God with Others

During one of my pregnancies, I was involved in leading a Bible study. This proved to be a wonderful way to hold myself accountable to search God's Word and really digest it. I still remember the book we studied, and some of the concepts I learned there were planted deeply in my soul. So even though "pregnancy brain" is a very real thing, God can overcome it and help us to grasp His precepts and principles and apply them to our lives.

Another good idea is to study the Word with your husband, if he is willing. Read passages on parenting, pray together, and commit your roles as Mom and Dad to the Lord. This will not only bring you individually closer to the Lord, but closer to one another as well.

Worship the Lord, Mama!

Four times now, pregnancy has been one of the most sanctifying seasons of my life. The Lord has brought sins to light that I had no idea were even an issue. He has walked me through intense times of laying down my pride, selfishness, self-pity, and insecurity. I have recognized my weakness and my need for Him during pregnancy more than almost any other season of life. And I am so thankful!

When God works in our lives, when He brings to light uncomfortable truths, it is a testimony of His great love for us. He could have abandoned us to our sins and allowed us to suffer the consequences of our foolish thinking (Romans 1:20–32). Instead, simply because we have chosen to follow His Son, He is molding us each day, shaping us more and more into His Son's image, and this is a beautiful thing (2 Corinthians 3:18). Thus He draws us to a place where, in love and adoration, we can see ever more clearly how wonderful He is!

ELLA
Mother of Five

Worship releases faith! No matter what our circumstances, when we stand firm on the promises of God, declaring His faithfulness and goodness, something shifts in the spiritual realm and in the depth of our soul, and we are able to mount up with wings like eagles, run and not grow weary, and dance upon our disappointments (Isaiah 40:31).

I have to admit, as much as I love singing praises to my beloved King, there have been times in my own life while carrying my five little bundles of joy that singing was just about the furthest thing from my mind. I certainly have missed many opportunities to exercise my faith through praising Him—especially in the valleys, where I often find myself during the first months of morning sickness, and in the desert places when I feel like I'm being stretched from all sides (and I'm not just talking about the skin on my stomach).

But the Lord ever so gently leads those who are with young (Isaiah 40:11), and He will meet us in our moments of desperation and weariness when we cry out to Him. He then shifts our gaze from the temporary to the eternal, and suddenly our whole perspective changes and we're reminded, "Weeping may tarry for the night, but joy comes with the morning" (Psalm 30:5).

Several studies have confirmed the many health benefits of singing. It's known to stimulate circulation, lower stress levels, release endorphins (the happy hormones), and help with muscle tension to name a few. Singing may also improve mental alertness and alleviate snoring.[1] But as we add to this physical list advantages from the spiritual dimension, mamas, we are onto something **really** good!

When we start to sing and praise Almighty God with our whole hearts, resisting the devil and meditating on the Lord's goodness, the enemy has no choice but to flee (James 4:7). The fog of doubt, fear, and self-pity that so easily clouds our minds simply evaporates as we worship the Lord. Through worship we remind ourselves of who He is, what He is capable of, and what **we** are not. There is no sweeter way to walk with Jesus than to rejoice continually in your utter dependence on Him.

However, the Lord often has to remind me to sing my songs on **both** sides of the Red Sea. It's easy to pull out the streamers and tambourines after the victory has been won, but what about during those times when we find ourselves right smack in the middle of a battle that, in the natural, looks completely hopeless? Songs of praise come easily when we're feeling good, but the refining of our character and faith often comes through trials and difficulty.

How the Lord must delight in the songs of His children when we declare our love and faith in the midst of the most challenging hardships! My husband and I have experienced our share of the fear and anxiety that often comes with childbearing. But oh, how we've witnessed, even in the delivery room, the Lord's surrounding us with songs of deliverance! Our hospital quarters have turned into such sweet sanctuaries of praise, even in the midst of great fear and pain. He has always provided us with just the right song to sing (or play on my husband's laptop) so that our spirits soar. The hospital staff can't say enough about the peacefulness in the room during these times.

I love the biblical depiction of Mary and her beautiful response to Gabriel's shocking baby announcement. She must have known immediately that this most certainly would be the eyebrow-raising talk of the town, but she didn't let that steal her joy and her confidence in God. She sang, "My soul magnifies the Lord, and my spirit rejoices in God my Savior" (Luke 1:46–47). May this be the cry of our hearts, and may we possess this attitude whether we are facing the unexpected or fighting the resentment of the mundane. He who has called us to motherhood is faithful, and He will do it.

3

Pregnancy and Marriage

*Two are better than one, because they have a good reward
for their toil. For if they fall, one will lift up his fellow.
But woe to him who is alone when he falls and has not
another to lift him up! Again, if two lie together, they keep
warm, but how can one keep warm alone? And though
a man might prevail against one who is alone, two will
withstand him—a threefold cord is not quickly broken.*
Ecclesiastes 4:9–12

"Hey, Babe, are you getting up?"

I was roused from sleep by the sound of my husband's voice
and his gentle hand on my shoulder. I could hear my 5:30
alarm going off, and I knew that if I wanted to make it to the
gym that day, I'd have to answer the call and leave behind my
nice, warm blankets. But that was the last thing my exhausted,
thirty-weeks-pregnant body wanted to do.

No sooner had I swung my legs over the edge of the bed than
the tears began to flow, and a deluge of pent-up discouragement
and frustration spilled out and into my husband's own tired ears.
"I slept so terribly last night, and my nerve pain is getting worse,
so I don't know if it's even worth it to try to go to the gym. On
top of that, I gained another five pounds the past two weeks, so
I don't think it's doing any good. And now I only have one pair
of workout pants that fit, and I'm pretty sure they're dirty ..."

The monologue continued as I tried to pull myself together enough to make it out the door. Finally, as I flopped down on the living room couch, holding one shoe in my hand, my sweet husband standing in front of me, all I could do was cry.

"Honey," he said, "I have no idea what to say. I've tried to encourage you, and I could tell you again that you look beautiful and that you're doing a great job, but that will only go so far."

I knew he was right. As much as I wanted in that moment to be coddled and complimented and cheered for again, that wasn't what I really needed.

These tearful bouts had been going on for weeks. Although I was carrying my third child, it was the first time I had experienced such deep emotional struggles connected to pregnancy. At times it all seemed too much to bear. The inability to control my emotions was stealing my joy and causing all kinds of insecurities to flare up more than they had in years. I was at my wit's end. I had tried reading Scripture, listening to podcasts, and playing worship music throughout the day. Yet day after day, I found myself trudging through an emotional bog I had no idea how to get out of.

That morning, as I looked up into Judah's face, I choked out in desperation, "Please, speak truth to me. I need to hear truth."

So he began speaking firmly, yet so tenderly, about the lies I was giving in to, and how I needed to stop listening to them and turn to Jesus. He reminded me that I *know* truth; I just needed to walk in it. He reminded me that my worth is in Christ, not in how my body looks. Okay, I was gaining weight, but that was supposed to happen because my body was home to the little life growing inside me.

There was nothing flowery about what Judah said. He wasn't trying to build my self-esteem or give me a pat on the back. He was lovingly exhorting me and even calling me out so that I wouldn't be trapped in this cycle of defeat.

It was exactly what I needed. From that day on, I kept a firm grasp on truth. The fog around my mind lifted, and joy began to flood back in. When the enemy's lies tried to come back, I could hear my husband's words in my head, reminding me not to slip back into wrong thinking but instead rest in Christ.

So I wiped my tears, gave Judah a smile, and waddled out the door to the gym.

The Gift of a Godly Husband

God has used Judah so many times to point me back to Himself. He has truly been my most faithful teammate and strongest encourager. I can't imagine walking through pregnancy (or life) without him. One thing I have learned, though, is that I have to *let* him be there for me. I must invite him in, with my words and demeanor. So I try to intentionally include Judah in every aspect of my pregnancy and welcome his input when he offers it.

During my first pregnancy, in the weeks before our son was born, Judah was reading a book (written by a Christian) about preparing to be a dad. Every once in a while I would read a chapter out loud to him so that we could glean some insights together about Judah's upcoming role as a father. After a couple of chapters, I started to feel growing indignation; something just didn't sit right with me about what we were reading.

One evening, after reading a particularly infuriating section, I stopped midsentence and exclaimed, "That is *just not true!*" As we talked through what was off about the book, we realized that its message seemed to be, "Dad, you're going to be a third wheel for a while. Baby takes priority, and you need to be okay with that. Just be there for Mom when she needs you—give her a hug and change the diapers."

I'm not saying everything in the book was terrible. The authors had some good, practical advice to offer. But much of its "wisdom" was based on human reasoning and experience rather than on God's Word and His design for the marriage relationship.

As women, we can so easily slip into a worldly mindset of prioritizing other things ahead of our marriage, *particularly* children. One reason is that the world is constantly telling women how pregnancy is all about Mom and the baby—making sure that *we* are comfortable, *we* are happy, *our* needs are being met. But pregnancy is *not* just about the mother and child. Your husband is just as much a parent to this child as you are, and he has an incredibly vital role to play in the child's life. He has the God-given responsibility of being the head of the home, and he is commanded to be actively involved in caring for and discipling his children (Ephesians 6:4). And this leadership role needs to be established from the moment you find out a little one will be joining your family.

The mother's role in carrying the child certainly takes a special grace and sensitivity to understand, and this is part of the husband's biblical role:

> *Husbands, live with your wives in an understanding way, showing honor to the woman as the weaker vessel, since they are heirs with you of the grace of life, so that your prayers may not be hindered. (1 Peter 3:7).*

Meanwhile, we are to honor and respect our husbands in every season of life, including pregnancy:

> *Wives, submit to your husbands, as is fitting in the Lord. (Colossians 3:18)*

> *Wives, be subject to your own husbands, so that even if some do not obey the word, they may be won without a word by the conduct of their wives. (1 Peter 3:1)*

I don't have a right to be snappy toward my husband or treat him in a dishonoring way just because of my hormones or a backache. And I can't assume that if I keep him out of the leadership role during my pregnancy that he will suddenly step up again once the baby arrives. God's truth is *always* true and *always* relevant, and it is *always* going to bring about greater love and strength in our marriage when I walk in obedience to the Lord by allowing my husband to be the leader God created him to be.

Marriage was instituted by God to manifest the gospel (Ephesians 5:21–33). As John and Nöel Piper write in their book *This Momentary Marriage*, "The meaning of marriage is the display of the covenant-keeping love between Christ and His people."[1] God's intent doesn't change with seasons or circumstances. There is never a time when a marriage is exempt from displaying the greater reality of Christ's relationship with the church. For this reason, the marriage relationship *must* remain our highest priority once children are in the picture.

Yes, things will change once a baby arrives. Yes, this baby will take up a huge amount of time and energy, especially from you, Mama. But what will ultimately help that child to thrive as an adult is to grow up witnessing what a godly marriage is supposed to look like, not by being the top priority in your life.

When we choose to obey God and live out marriage as He intended it to be, our marriage becomes a marvel to those watching. When a husband and wife love and serve one another even when the family is changing or circumstances become difficult, the gospel shines boldly through that family and becomes attractive to a lost and dying world. When a woman, even in the more difficult moments of pregnancy, chooses to joyfully obey God's direction for being a wife and mother, you can be sure it will not go unnoticed.

Created to Be a Team

In sports, a team is a group of individuals with different talents, skills, and responsibilities who work together to achieve a common goal. For the team to be successful, every member of the team has to know the playbook and understand his or her assignment on every play. The players must communicate constantly, always give their best effort, and hold one another accountable. And every player must make decisions (on and off the field) that put the good of the team ahead of their selfish desires.

Does this sound like your home? After all, God designed marriage to function as a team. Think about it: Husband and wife both bring different talents and skills to the marriage, and each of them has unique roles and responsibilities within the family. Both need to study the playbook (the Bible), listen to the head coach (Jesus), and follow His instructions. Both have to make the decision every day to put the other's needs first and selflessly serve one another in love. If both of them make a genuine effort to communicate daily and work toward the same goals, husband and wife can accomplish far more together as a team than either one could ever hope to achieve by themselves.

This is true during pregnancy too. In sports, if one player tries to hog the ball and make all the plays, the team suffers. If you try to do all the planning and preparation for baby's arrival or keep your husband at arm's length because you don't think he'll understand when you're feeling emotional, the marriage will suffer. True, your husband doesn't get to carry "the ball" during these nine months, but he can "block" for you and provide valuable support and encouragement as your teammate, confidante, and number one fan. And don't forget, as team captain, it's his job to help you stay focused on Jesus.

Some husbands take a lot of flak about being clueless or uncaring when it comes to their pregnant wives. But I don't believe this is always (or completely) the husband's fault. If his wife is not proactive to involve him in the pregnancy or does not communicate her specific needs, then we can't put all the blame on him. Sometimes, he might simply be unsure about what he can do to help or encourage his wife. After all, it's true that with all the hormonal activity and physical changes happening to our bodies, we moms-to-be can be a *little bit* more emotional than usual. So it's only natural that our husbands should feel helpless at times or confused about what we need at any given moment.

Men do tend to have a "fix it" mentality; when they encounter a problem, their first response is to try to fix it. A number of times during my pregnancies, if it was clear I was struggling with something, Judah would try to help by speaking clear, strong truth to me—often when I would rather not hear it. I knew he was trying to be helpful and a good leader, but everything in me wanted to be offended because he obviously didn't understand what I was feeling. Sometimes, I just wanted him to say, "I'm so sorry," and wrap his arms around me and let me cry, even when I also knew that coddling would get me nowhere and might only cause more trouble. (Um, I might have—*cough, cough*—learned that from experience.)

But as I respectfully listened and humbly accepted my husband's advice, the Lord would often open an opportunity to approach Judah with how he could best encourage me in different situations. Over time we have both learned how to serve one another better. Judah has learned not to immediately resort to fix-it mode, and I have learned not to be defensive when he reminds me of God's truth. And each pregnancy has grown us closer together because of this.

Consider Him First

I mentioned that marriage works best when each spouse puts the other first. As expectant mothers, we often hear that in our condition we need to think of ourselves and put *our* needs first, but this is just not true. Jesus praised the example of the poor widow who, out of her poverty, gave everything she had to God (Mark 12:41–44). When Jesus was dying on the cross, He was still thinking about other people (John 19:26–27; Luke 23:42–43). He set the ultimate example of laying down one's rights to put others first, even to the point of death.

When I keep Jesus at the forefront of my mind and my heart, serving and loving my husband becomes a joy in every circumstance. I have the opportunity to serve and love my husband unlike any other person on earth, and when I make the effort to do that a time when the world says I should be taking care of my own needs, you can be sure the effort is noticed—by him and by others.

As your pregnancy progresses and becomes more and more physically challenging, you can still maintain a mindset of putting your husband's needs before your own. You might have to be a bit more creative and think outside the box. But as you seek the Lord and ask Him how to best love your husband, the Lord will give you wisdom and inspiration.

Here are some ideas I've tried that have helped to make my husband feel loved and involved during these nine months.

Talk with Him

Our tendency is to talk to another woman about our prenatal difficulties. But talking them over with your husband as well is a wonderful way to bring him into what you're walking through. He may not always understand right away, so you may be forced to employ your best communication skills along with humility, patience, and understanding. But whether he shows it or not, I have no doubt he will be honored that you want to share this with him.

I have to be very careful with my tone when I approach my husband about these issues. If I am whiny or seem accusatory in any way (as in "You're not ..." or "I wish you would ..." or "Why can't you ...") it puts him on the defensive, and he has the tendency to then pull away. But if I come seeking advice, asking for prayer, and being willing to hear what he has to say, it endears me to him. And almost without fail, his compassionate and comforting side emerges and he invites me to cry on his shoulder or simply snuggle in his arms. This is imperative preparation for the labor process, which we will go into in a later chapter.

Serve Him

One of the wisest things my mother told me before my wedding was that there would be times I wouldn't feel like loving my husband sexually, but that putting his needs above my own in that way would speak volumes to him. This wasn't a problem in the early days of our marriage, but I was greatly put to the test in this way during pregnancy. At first, it was the twenty-four-hour nausea. Later, it was the growing belly, the terrible nerve and back pain, and the lack of sleep. I felt *so* justified in all the reasons I wanted to say no. But those times I chose to deny myself and love my husband in that way, we were drawn closer together. And he would often lay down *his* desires to serve me. He could see that I was making an effort to meet his sexual needs, and in turn, he would go out of his way to love me in the ways that were most meaningful to me.

This is not to say that I don't sometimes ask to take a rain check. But because of my willingness at other times, he doesn't take it as a slight, because he knows I truly desire to honor and love him as best I can.

[Note: I'm not addressing here situations in which physical intimacy is considered unsafe due to complications with the pregnancy. In such circumstances, use the time to talk and pray with your husband about how God might want to grow you closer during this unique season.]

In marriage, it is so easy to justify selfishness. It can even be done under the guise of spirituality. The husband might be thinking, *She should be respecting me by doing what is most important to me,* while at the same time the wife is thinking, *He is commanded to live with me in an understanding way!* When both of us are focused on ourselves, there is more conflict and tension in the home. But when each of us is focused on serving the other, it just *works.* We stop being so focused on our own desires, and it becomes a delight to love and serve each other as we are commanded to do out of obedience to the Lord. As Jesus said in Matthew 7:12, "Whatever you wish that others would do to you, do also to them."

Seek Him Out

There are few things that will endear a husband to his wife more than when she seeks his advice and genuinely takes it into consideration. This is a display of respect and trust in his counsel and a way of showing him you truly care about what he has to say.

During pregnancy, it may not seem that your husband would have much advice to offer, at least in practical things like which creams are best for preventing stretch marks or which support stockings might be the best investment. However, he might have insight into the emotional, physical, or spiritual aspects of pregnancy that you're not seeing immediately. Just because he has never carried a baby to term doesn't mean he has nothing to offer regarding the principle of the matter.

Consider that the apostle Paul wrote quite extensively in Scripture about marriage, parenting, and other areas of life that he personally had no experience in. Yet how silly would it be of us to disregard his teaching in family matters just because he was a lifelong bachelor? Yes, Paul was inspired by God to write these things, but we are inhabited by the same Spirit and have the same wisdom available to us. As he wrote in 2 Timothy

3:16–17, "All Scripture is breathed out by God and profitable for teaching, for reproof, for correction, and for training in righteousness." If your husband is offering any kind of advice based on principles found in the Bible, then it is profitable for you and may be exactly what you need to hear.

Spend Time with Him

If you are expecting your first child, remember that these are the last days you and your husband will have at home with just the two of you for a long time. This is by no means a bad thing, but do realize that your life is about to become very different. There is no better way of preparing for your new little one than by cherishing the time you and your husband have together as just the two of you.

From the early days of my first pregnancy, Judah and I prayed together, read books together, and spent a lot of time seeking counsel from wise and experienced parents. I asked Judah's opinion on crib and stroller choices, and even though we didn't always agree, when we went with his first choice, often I was later glad we had. We were able to take some shorter getaways, and we tried to be intentional about doing fun, pregnancy-safe activities together that were out of the ordinary.

Just ask and the Lord will give you wisdom as a couple to know what this might look like for you. For now, here are a few suggestions:

- Go on walks together. It's a great way to connect while getting some low-impact exercise.
- Take a mini vacation. Even if it's not that far away, just getting away from your usual environment can be refreshing while removing distractions.
- Read pregnancy and parenting books together.
- Pray together about the details of your pregnancy, delivery, and preparation for becoming parents.

I love how Martin Luther said it all those years ago: "There is no more lovely, friendly, or charming relationship, communion, or company than a good marriage." As you commit to investing in your marriage to the glory of God during your pregnancy, He will honor it in more ways than you may ever know.

Testimony from a Faithful Wife (and Mama)

ELSJE
Mother of Three

I was around thirty-nine weeks pregnant when we had a slightly unpleasant visit with our midwife. I was measuring pretty small and hadn't gained a significant amount of weight. Now, this **was** my first pregnancy, and I am only about the size of a large child myself, so taking these things into account, it wasn't anything unusual. But the midwife showed a bit of concern and talked about my having to get some tests done.

As a first-time mom, this sent me into quite the spell of worry. No mom wants to hear that her baby might be at risk. I was quite the mess, and yet my husband remained calm and collected. At first I was almost upset with him that he refused to join in my anxiety. How dare he be so optimistic and cool while I was clearly unraveling!

However, as he remained undisturbed by it all, I remembered that I needed to honor him and the position he had taken of not calling every doctor in the Northern Hemisphere to set up 4D ultrasounds to make sure the baby was okay. He was simply trusting God and showing me that I needed to trust Him as well. It would have been so easy for me to instead try to convince him that he was not the pregnant one, he should listen to me, and we immediately should Google all the possible things that might be wrong with our child.

There are definitely times when it's appropriate for the pregnant mom to seek additional medical help. In our situation, though, there really was nothing out of the ordinary or alarming about the circumstances. Nevertheless, I needed my husband to point this out to me, and I needed to honor his position in order to see it. Our sweet baby girl was born two weeks later—lovely, pink, and perfectly healthy.

While not without controversy in our egalitarian age, the concept of showing honor and respect isn't new to most Christian women. Respecting your husband doesn't always come easy, but it can seem to come more naturally when you and your spouse are on the same page, walking through the same thing together. For instance, when the bank account runs dangerously low—not an uncommon experience in the early days of many marriages—you both need to seek God for grace and exert faith in Him together. You are both, after all, in the exact same financial position, so honoring your husband (and maybe even showing a little kindness toward him) should come pretty easily to you.

Of course, pregnancy is a bit different. Although you are both expecting, just one of you is pregnant. Your husband is not experiencing firsthand the morning sickness, indigestion, sleeplessness, and the emotional roller-coaster. He is sharing in the joy and anticipation of the new life but is spared the watermelon tummy, microscopic bladder, and odd hankerings. This is a massive grace of God. Imagine if both of you were undergoing these immense physical, hormonal, and emotional changes at the same time!

The thing is, pregnancy provides a unique opportunity for you to show that same honor and respect to your husband, even when he's not walking through exactly what you are. He may be blissfully ignorant of what it feels like to be pregnant, but that doesn't make him less worthy of your honor and respect. He is still your husband. He is still your head, placed in this position by the Lord God Himself (Ephesians 5:23).

As I look back on that situation involving the midwife and my first child, I see that it was an opportunity to learn that even though my husband didn't entirely understand all that I was going through, he was still uniquely gifted and positioned by God to lead me through it.

4

Pregnancy and Family

Behold, children are a heritage from the LORD,
the fruit of the womb a reward.
Psalm 127:3

I remember clearly the day my then-one-year-old son, Jude, felt his baby sister kick for the first time inside me. As his little hand rested on my belly, he waited (uncharacteristically) patiently for any sign of movement. When finally he was rewarded with a nudge, Jude looked up at me with surprise written all over his tiny face. I told him that was his little sister, and he broke into a huge smile.

We had been preparing him for the baby's arrival since the day we found out she had reservations at Chez Mama. Jude quickly caught on that baby was in mommy's tummy and would often mention it to me, patting me gently. When we learned she was a girl, he would exuberantly exclaim, "Hi, Jenesis!" to my growing baby bump. Hugs for her became a common occurrence, and he would lavish her (or rather, my belly) with kisses. We figured that if we brought big brother into the excitement early on, he was more likely to be just as excited once she arrived. And we weren't disappointed.

When Jude met Jenesis for the first time, he was clearly filled with awe. He sat next to me and looked at her little toes and little fingers and smiled shyly as we told him this was the baby he had been talking to and loving on from the outside. He would stand beside her cradle and just stare at her and tell her, "I love you," in the sweetest voice. He would ask to see her every morning when he woke up. After nine months of our talking to him every day about the baby and preparing him to welcome this addition to our family, he was overjoyed when she arrived. And watching their interaction is still one of the most precious things in my life.

A couple of years later we had the joy of seeing Jude and Jenesis welcome another small person into our family. Jude was thrilled from the day we told him I was expecting and would often talk to Jenesis about the baby, pointing to my tummy and explaining in his toddler way about a new sibling while Jenesis stared incredulously. She clearly had no idea what he was talking about. Jude loved coming to my appointments and hearing the baby's heartbeat. He sat with wide eyes as he watched the ultrasound that revealed we were having another baby girl. I was observing Jenesis quietly as the months went by, and even though I knew she couldn't quite grasp the concept, I prayed that she would welcome the baby the same way Jude had welcomed Jenesis.

One day in my third trimester, I walked in the front door after being gone awhile. Jenesis ran up to me, looking from my face to my tummy, and a light suddenly came on for her. "Baby! I kiss baby!" she exclaimed. I knelt down and she put her head down by my tummy. From that day on, her excitement never waned, and both she and Jude welcomed their newborn sister with genuine delight.

Preparing for Two (or Three or Four)

I've talked to many expectant mothers who are nervous about how their children will respond to a new sibling. If you are preparing for a second or third (or fourth) child, I'm sure you've had similar thoughts. *How in the world do we prepare for this? What practical steps should we take? Do we expect the best or prepare for the worst—or both? Will my other children feel neglected because I need to spend so much time with the baby? Will they understand that my love for them hasn't changed even though my time and attention are divided?*

Our desire as parents is to have children that love each other from the start, so we feel the pressure of wanting to get this *right*, bringing the new child home to siblings who are smitten and who want to protect their younger brother or sister from any harm. Experienced moms know it requires effort. We also know that we can't do it in our own strength. Because all children are sinful and in need of Jesus, we must pray and trust Him to build that selfless love between our children, to give us wisdom in fostering this even before the new sibling enters the world.

Practically Loving Your "External" Children

A friend of mine who was pregnant with her second child expressed to me the struggle of knowing how to care for her first while in the midst of morning sickness. She was working through how to practically love and serve her son when she could barely get out of bed.

I've experienced this too.

You feel that all you can do is lie on the couch, but your little son needs lunch and asks for food that makes you gag.

You're spending most of your time on the bathroom floor, but your daughter wants to go to the park.

Your little one wants sit on your lap to read books, but your growing belly takes up too much space.

It's no wonder we fall into the trap of worrying that bringing another child into the family will make the others feel less loved and cared for. This is not to say there won't be an adjustment period. It may be that you will walk through some struggles with jealousy, as some families do. But take heart that God desires unity within your family, just as He desires unity within His church. And when you seek Him and ask how you can encourage and prepare your kids to welcome the new arrival, He will be faithful to give you the wisdom you need to navigate changes in the family dynamics.

Again, It Takes Intentionality

It can be easy to subconsciously put our children on the back burner while dealing with the side effects of pregnancy. We might not even realize we're doing it at first until we begin to see changes in our children's behavior, their words, and their attitudes. (I know this from experience, by the way.) The last thing we want to do is cause insecurity in our young children, and the best way we can avoid that is to continually look for little ways to serve and love them. How we do this may look very different from those times when we're not pregnant. But children are quick to see the intent of a mother's heart, which is ultimately more important than the details of *how* we serve and love them each day.

Keep in mind that when you cultivate a heart of service toward your children, putting their needs and wants ahead of your own, you are ultimately doing it for Jesus. When He returns, Jesus will gather all the nations and separate the righteous from the unrighteous, and He will say to the righteous:

> *"Come, you who are blessed by my Father, inherit*
> *the kingdom prepared for you from the foundation of*
> *the world. For I was hungry and you gave me food, I*
> *was thirsty and you gave me drink, I was a stranger*

and you welcomed me, I was naked and you clothed me, I was sick and you visited me, I was in prison and you came to me" (Matthew 25:34–36).

When the righteous say they don't remember doing these things for Jesus, He will reply, "As you did it to one of the least of these my brothers, you did it to me" (v. 40).

We do many of these things for our young children day in and day out. We feed them, clothe them, comfort them, and care for them when they are sick. A tired mom can sometimes feel that her ministrations are insignificant, but in God's eyes, we are living out the calling on our lives. When we do these things with joy and purpose, we are doing the most important, spiritual thing we can be doing in that moment.

So when it is all you can do to just lift your head off the pillow, and your child wants that one thing that makes your stomach most queasy, you have to remember the big picture. When you put your children's needs ahead of your own, you are preaching the gospel to them. And they will, Lord willing, one day follow your example.

My son is very outgoing and craves time with other people, so it was pretty hard on him when I was sick during my second pregnancy. Because I was his sole means of personal interaction for so much of the day, I had to get creative. When all I could do was lie on the couch, I had him snuggle up next to me and read books or watch "Silly Songs with Larry" (sometimes over and over again). I tried to keep healthy snack items on hand that he really enjoyed (and my stomach could handle being around). I was required to snack throughout the day, so he would snack with me. We spent time outdoors, sitting in the grass and watching the cars pass by our home. When I was up to it, we would take short walks around the neighborhood, pointing out all the doggies and greeting everyone we saw. Those simple, yet intentional acts meant the world to him.

That difficult pregnancy ended up being a sweet season of building my relationship with my son, and it laid for him the foundation of knowledge that bringing another child into the family would in no way change my love for him.

Inviting Your Kids Into the Joy

I was warned many times to prepare for a negative reaction from little Jude when his baby sister came, and I was often asked with apprehension how we thought he would respond to sharing his parents with a sibling.

As we thought and prayed about it and sought advice from our parents and others, we became more and more convinced that if we made an effort to bring Jude into the joy of welcoming a new baby, we could expect that he would respond in kind. Of course, we were prepared for whatever the reaction might be, knowing that it really is hard for some kids. But after months of setting this before him as an exciting, wonderful thing, we fully anticipated that Jude would fall in love with his little sister.

Did it happen? Yes!

Has it been perfect? No.

Because sin and sin natures are part of the equation, no relationship between two humans will be perfect this side of heaven. With each new addition to the family, there are new layers of selfishness to deal with. But we have seen prayer after prayer answered as we've watched our children interact these past few years.

Solomon wrote, "Behold, children are a heritage from the LORD, the fruit of the womb a reward" (Psalm 127:3). This is the message we need to convey to all of our children, that every new life that enters the world—and this family—is a precious gift from God. This must taught both through our words and our attitudes. But some parents are so nervous about how their older child will react to a new sibling that they hardly mention it before the birth. All this does is set the child up for an even *greater* shock when one day Mom is in the hospital and snuggling a new rival for her attention.

You've probably heard stories of once-sweet children who suddenly became terrors when they found themselves sharing a mom and dad they previously had all to themselves. This is obviously the last thing you want for your older child. You know the transition won't be perfect, but is there something you can do practically to prepare your child, perhaps even help them to be excited for the baby to come?

Yes.

Start with Prayer

The very first step in any major life transition is to go to the Lord in prayer. God's Word makes it so clear that He loves to answer our prayers abundantly. Think about the men and women considered to have been heroes of the Christian faith. There's one thing they all had in common: prayer. These people prayed about everything, big and small, and God answered.

When we pray according to the will of God, we can be sure He will answer affirmatively. We know, for example, that He greatly desires unity and love among believers (Philippians 1:27; Ephesians 4:1–3), so pray this for your children. As Psalm 133:1 reads, "Behold, how good and pleasant it is when brothers dwell in unity!"

Your family dynamics might not look exactly like you thought they would, but in the end they can be better than you ever imagined. When we are purposeful about praying for our children and diligently seeking God's Word for wisdom on how to train and prepare them to be followers of Christ, He will give us everything we need. Then we can look forward in hope to what Proverbs 22:6 says: "Train up a child in the way he should go; even when he is old he will not depart from it."

What About Your Extended Family?

Before moving on, I want to share a few brief thoughts on involving your extended family when you're preparing to have a baby.

When we found out we were pregnant for the first time, we wasted no time letting our family know. They knew that we weren't even sure we would be able to have children, so sharing the news right away only enhanced our joy. They were all elated, to say the least! One of my younger sisters began researching all things pregnancy, and she would often inform me about the current stage of the unborn baby's development, what I should and shouldn't be doing, and how I could best prepare for labor. Everyone shared their suggestions for baby names and eagerly awaited the news as to whether it was a boy or a girl.

Because my family lives in Thailand and Judah's in Mongolia, we knew that if we stayed in Colorado for the birth that very few of our immediate family would be able to be present when Jude was born. So we decided to go to them! I was thirty-four weeks pregnant when we packed our bags and flew halfway around the world to Chiang Mai, Thailand. Judah's mom and youngest brother flew in from Mongolia to be with us too. It was such a special time of being together, and they all told us many times how thankful and honored they were that we went out of our way (literally) to include them.

For some, like us, involving family has only been a joy. But I know many people who have wrestled through circumstances involving more difficult or complex family dynamics. When extended family is dysfunctional, when ties have been broken or strained, it can be very difficult to know how best to share the arrival of a new family member.

Judah and I talked not long ago with a wonderful couple preparing to welcome their first child, a girl. One of their siblings had chosen a sinful lifestyle, and the couple were wrestling with what that sibling's relationship with their child would look like as she grew. Maybe for you the difficulty is a parent who is critical of every decision you make, constantly micromanaging and offering unsolicited opinions. Perhaps one of you has an estranged father or a brother or sister who is an outspoken unbeliever.

Whatever the case may be, God has created this new life growing inside of you, and He has a perfect plan. He chose the family this child is being born into, and His choice was no accident (Acts 17:26–27). He might use this child to bring unity to a family that was once fractured and broken, though it may be years down the road. Think of Joseph, who was sold into slavery by his family. Yet ultimately God used him to save his family from a devastating famine (Genesis 37–45). So begin to pray now for your precious little one, that he or she will be used to deepen bonds, heal wounds, and soften hearts.

This new life that is coming into the world has the potential to be used in amazing ways. God will surely bless you as you seek Him and His will for your child. Walk faithfully in the wisdom He delights to give to you when you delight yourself in Him!

CAROL BETH

Mother of Eight

I woke up in the middle of the night with a pain in my abdomen more intense than anything I'd ever experienced. It wasn't unusual to be awakened during the night by noises outside our apartment building or by the cries of one of our seven children. My husband is not a very sound sleeper, so he often got up to respond to the needs of a little one or, peering out the window, pray for those making a commotion outside the bar across the street. This time, however, I tried to avoid waking him as I climbed out of bed, crawled into the bathroom, and retched violently. Eventually, I went back to bed, but the excruciating pain didn't subside. So, in tears, I reluctantly woke my husband.

Living in Ulaanbaatar, Mongolia, one of the biggest challenges we faced was how to handle medical emergencies. As in many post-communist countries, Mongolia's hospitals and clinics lacked equipment and supplies and their medical personnel were often undertrained. The infant mortality rate in Mongolia was exceptionally high, and quality care for pre-term babies was virtually nonexistent.

I was twenty-four weeks pregnant.

So my husband and I prayed together and waited a few hours before calling our friend, an American doctor who had been serving in Mongolia with his wife since shortly after the democratic revolution opened the country in the early 1990s. By the time he arrived, about a half hour after our call, the intensity of my pain had subsided to a dull ache. After examining me, he suggested we visit the maternity hospital, which housed one of only a few outdated ultrasound machines in the country.

The ultrasound confirmed that our baby was okay and showed no evidence of any damage. We were thankful for the good news, yet still curious about what might have caused such an intense pain. Since then, we've come to believe it was most likely a kidney stone. I've overheard conversations about which is worse, the pain of labor or a kidney stone. After experiencing the pain of labor with seven different deliveries, I only know I would certainly choose labor over the pain I experienced that night.

After a few days, I was feeling fairly normal again, with the exception of ongoing, increasing contractions. Almost any activity would stimulate contractions, so my husband decided (after a lot of research) it would be best for me to be on bed rest.

I am blessed to have a husband who is extremely good at protecting and caring for his family. Not only did he take on a greater role with meal preparation and household management, but he also enlisted our children to help out. He impressed upon the children the importance of doing everything possible to keep Mom in bed and not cause extra stress. He admonished them to be a blessing to one another, doing their best to avoid quarrels and to keep the house peaceful and orderly. At the time, our oldest child was almost fourteen, and the youngest was two. They all offered assistance and expressed concern to the extent that each of them was able to understand the importance of keeping Mom from going into labor too early.

I was blessed by my family as they joyfully served and cared for me, but it was difficult for me not to struggle with feelings of discouragement and guilt for not taking care of them as I usually would. It was quite humbling to allow the children to do things for me. I also had to be careful not to be critical of their efforts to do things that I might have done differently. One of the things that was hardest for me during bed rest was being separated from the family activity in the kitchen and living area of our apartment. When the children realized that they could encourage me just by being near me, they began to bring their schoolbooks and toys into the bedroom to keep me company.

As the weeks went by with no improvement, my husband called the doctor of our mission organization to get his opinion. After a long night of phone calls, it was decided that the best course of action was an immediate air evacuation, which ended up being the very next day. Unaware of this, I awakened while the children were still sleeping, and I went out to sit in our living room recliner. The quiet, dimly lit room was decorated for the celebration of our daughter's twelfth birthday later that day. My heart was filled with joy as I spent time alone with the Lord, thanking Him for His abundant blessings, for His steadfast provision, for each of our sweet children, for a loving and protective husband, and for parents who were faithfully following Jesus and living for His glory.

Sometime in the stillness of the morning, before sunrise, my husband snuck into the room and shared the news that I would be taken by an air ambulance later that day to Beijing, China. My heart was still no longer as I became overwhelmed by anxious thoughts. *Not on our daughter's birthday! Not today!* I asked if we could tell them not to come, but the doctor had informed him that once the mission organization had been made aware of my situation, legally there was no other option. I was to be flown to the safety of a hospital where, if they could not stop the contractions, there would be a better chance of survival for the baby.

As the Lord so graciously provides for His children, my parents had already planned on spending several weeks with our family in Mongolia, and they happened to be there as all this was unfolding. When the children and my parents had awoken and gathered, we told them about the unexpected surprise that would make this birthday different from what we had planned. We did our best to make the remainder of the day special for our daughter and to help the children have an attitude of thanksgiving for the way the Lord had provided care and protection for Mom and their unborn sibling.

So we prayed together and talked about our expectations for what would happen next. Our birthday girl helped me pack my suitcase, and though it was sad for her to know we were leaving, she very graciously accepted the added responsibilities of helping Grandpa and Grandma while we were gone.

My parents were scheduled to return to Colorado about the same time our family had been planning to fly to Thailand three weeks later, but due to the sudden change of plans, they extended their visas to remain in Mongolia with our seven children and then fly with them to meet us in Thailand, where we still hoped to deliver our baby as planned.

The medical evacuation team arrived mid-afternoon, and I was prepped and loaded into the back of an old Russian ambulance. The whole experience was surreal and uncomfortable, but the worst part for me was looking up from the stretcher as they pushed me into the vehicle to see our children watching and waving from the apartment window. I didn't know if any of them were crying, but I sure was.

After a few days in Beijing, the doctors were able to bring the contractions under control, and my husband and I were able to fly to Thailand as planned, where we met my parents and the children several weeks later, right before Christmas. On January 2, we celebrated the safe arrival of a perfectly healthy little girl. She was immediately embraced and loved by her older sisters and brothers, who understood that our gracious and merciful heavenly Father had provided and protected this precious gift to our family.

As I reflect on this experience, I realize how graciously the Lord provided for me through my family. Yes, it was difficult for me to release control of managing the household and allow my husband and children to take over chores that I was used to doing in my own way. I struggled to receive the beautiful gift that my family was giving me; it wasn't easy for me to lie in another room, thinking about all the things that needed to be done. I am so thankful now to realize that the Lord used this season to refine me and lead me into a place of deeper trust in Him, while providing my children and husband a beautiful opportunity to love and serve one another.

5

Pregnancy and Fear

"You keep him in perfect peace whose mind is stayed on you, because he trusts in you. Trust in the LORD forever, for the LORD GOD is an everlasting rock."
Isaiah 26:3–4

I was thirty-seven weeks pregnant with my third child, almost into the home stretch, when a routine prenatal exam suddenly wasn't so routine. Instead of the baby's growth being right on track as at every previous appointment, she suddenly appeared to be measuring two weeks behind. I could sense the concern my midwife was trying to conceal as she told me she was ordering an ultrasound just to check on everything.

A few hours later, I found myself lying in a dark room while an ultrasound technician probed my belly to get a more accurate measurement of the baby. As I lay on the table, I searched the face of the tech, commanding my heart to be still. *Oh Lord, please help this baby to be okay,* I prayed silently. They determined she was measuring smaller than she should be and scheduled me for a specialized ultrasound and more extensive monitoring, sending me home with repeated reminders to call should I feel any decrease in movement.

Although everyone was very calm and professional, their urgency and concern was almost palpable. And I knew I had a choice: Would I give in to the fear that was already threatening to overwhelm me? Or would I keep my eyes focused on Jesus, the creator and sustainer of the child in my womb?

The next couple of weeks were filled with more ultrasounds, more monitoring, and more pressing into Jesus. Even during labor there were multiple times when fear came knocking. But each time the temptation arose, I was reminded by my husband or a timely passage of Scripture that God is sovereign and fully in control. And as we welcomed our little girl into the world, we could testify to the fact that God's peace, not fear, surrounded us.

The temptation to take fear's bait is ever present for an expectant mom.

Should I be having that pain?

I don't feel as nauseated today—does that mean something?

When was the last time I felt him kick?

Do I have what it takes to care for more than one child?

What if something goes wrong during labor?

What if I go into labor right here, right now?!?

Something is stirred in a mother's heart for the child she's carrying: God-given love and a ferocious instinct to protect this child at any cost. So much is out of Mom's control when a little one is developing inside her womb, and often all she can do is wait. And pray. And wait some more. In these times of waiting, thinking, and preparing, the temptation to fear can be around any turn. The enemy of our souls knows that a mother is so vulnerable and susceptible to fear if she's not constantly on guard against it.

Generally speaking, God created women to be more expressive emotionally than men. This trait can add depth and richness to our lives and the lives of our families. However, problems arise when we have a difficult time keeping our emotions under control. This is especially hard when we're undergoing hormonal changes, and it is all too easy, commonplace even, to excuse the occasional emotional outburst during pregnancy. But you will find no place in Scripture that excuses us to act upon any fleshly instinct we may have, no matter what the situation.

We are called to "walk in a manner worthy of the Lord, fully pleasing to Him" (Colossians 1:10). Whenever we are tempted to be sullen, grumpy, frustrated, irritable, anxious, or given to self-pity, we need to stop and ask ourselves, *Will acting this way be fully pleasing to the Lord?* If the answer is no, then it's something we can't give in to. Of course, in and of our own strength, it's impossible not to give in to wrong emotions at some level. Believe me, I know this from personal experience. We may be able to fight them for a while, but there will come a point when we'll cave under pressure and act on them.

But this is where the beautiful, transforming power of the gospel comes in! Scripture says, "His divine power has granted to us all things that pertain to life and godliness, through the knowledge of him who called us to his own glory and excellence" (2 Peter 1:3). In Christ, you and I *do* have everything we need to speak, act, and think in a way that brings glory to God. Our job is to believe that His grace is with us, even if our emotions are telling us something else. When we submit our emotional lives to the Holy Spirit's control, He *will* give us everything we need to walk in a manner that glorifies Him.

I battled the stronghold of fear through much of my childhood. I began having panic attacks when I was seven years old, and I felt physically ill any time I even thought of anything bad that might happen to me or someone I loved. But shortly after I was married, the Lord really began to deal with this area of my life. And by His grace, I was able to surrender my fears to Him. This was a process of daily speaking truth to myself and choosing to walk in the promises in Scripture rather than giving in to feelings of fear as they came (2 Timothy 1:7).

I experienced so much freedom as a result, and I praise Him for that! What I didn't realize, however, was that with children would come a whole new level of sanctification and transformation in this area. I had no idea just how strongly the battle would rage within my mind and heart between seemingly overwhelming fear and the rock-solid truth of God's Word.

Most of us are familiar with these verses and others like them:

The LORD is my light and my salvation; whom shall I fear? The LORD is the stronghold of my life; of whom shall I be afraid? (Psalm 27:1)

Even though I walk through the valley of the shadow of death, I will fear no evil, for you are with me (Psalm 23:4).

But do we actually take their "no fear" message to heart? How often do we practically apply these truths to our everyday lives? So often we treat these passages as lovely poetry or true in principle, but when it comes down to it, many of us don't truly believe these promises apply in our situation. When fear comes knocking at your nursery door, do you immediately take the thought captive and make it obedient to the Lord (2 Corinthians 10:5)? Or do you surrender to the anxiety that so easily entangles as it wreaks havoc on your heart and mind (Proverbs 29:25; Hebrews 12:1)?

Looking back on my journey, I can identify several key moments when the choice lay before me: Was I going to trust my feelings or my God? Fear might have felt like the logical response to my circumstances, but I knew in the deepest part of my being that if I looked to the Lord, I would find the freedom from fear He promises. I also knew that if I did choose the path of fear, I was basically saying that I didn't *really* believe what God says in His Word.

I can tell you from personal experience that if you choose to trust God, He will come through every time. But it's not always easy. In fact, it sometimes feels as though you're having to fight against everything your mind and body are telling you to do. At such times, reach out to the Lord. Cling to Him and ask for His help, for He is always faithful.

You may not realize just how much you cling to fear (as if being afraid or anxious could do anything to change your present circumstance). After you've spent years giving in to fear and anxiety, learning to trust God requires a complete change of mindset that doesn't happen overnight. But as you choose to submit this area of your life to His care, your fear will gradually be replaced by an unshakeable peace that can only come from God.

What Is Fear?

After identifying an area of fearfulness or worry in your life, you must then recognize it for what it is—a lack of faith in God. Fear turns your eyes away from Him and onto your circumstances and all the "what ifs" out there. It causes doubt. At minimum, fear is a distraction that will keep you from drawing near to God, and this, in essence, is sin. We read time and again throughout Scripture the *command* not to be afraid (Deuteronomy 31:6; Joshua 8:1; Isaiah 43:1; Matthew 10:31; etc.). And what is the reason we are not to fear in all these verses? Because God loves us and is with us.

There is only one kind of fear that is good: the fear of the Lord. This fear drives away all others. This fear is an awe, a deep reverence, an awareness that He is far above us, that He is the Creator and Upholder of the universe, that nothing is outside of His realm of control, and that our lives are in His hands. As Nancy DeMoss Wolgemuth put it, the fear of the Lord is "a deep sense of reverence and awe from knowing we are in the presence of true greatness. The fear of the Lord is that constant, conscious sense of the presence of God."[1]

When we choose to look at any other fear through the lens of Scripture and a right understanding of who God is, all lesser fears cannot and will not remain:

> *In the fear of the LORD one has strong confidence, and his children will have a refuge. The fear of the LORD is a fountain of life, that one may turn away from the snares of death. (Proverbs 14:26–27)*

> *The fear of the LORD leads to life, and whoever has it rests satisfied; he will not be visited by harm. (Proverbs 19:23)*

> *The fear of man lays a snare, but whoever trusts in the LORD is safe. (Proverbs 29:25)*

Being firmly established in the fear of the Lord is the first step to becoming free from all other fears that would seek to keep you in their oppressive grip.

Beware of Isolation

One of the most effective tactics the enemy uses to try to get us to dwell on our fears is by making you and me think we are the only ones dealing with these fears. The longer we keep our fears in the dark, the more dangerous they become, implanting themselves in our minds and poisoning our thoughts. We don't want to voice them because we are concerned that others might think we're silly, or that they will be more likely to happen if we speak them, or any number of lies the enemy tries to get us to believe.

One day, early in my first pregnancy, I had been feeling quite crampy and was battling the fear of a miscarriage. I decided to tell Judah what was going on in my mind and heart. When I confessed my fear to him, he was able to point me back to the Lord and pray with me, asking the Lord to help me place those fears—and our baby—in His loving and capable hands. Afterward, those fears were dispelled, and any time during the pregnancy that fear would begin to arise, I could go back to that day, remembering the peace that came from casting my cares upon my heavenly Father.

When we confess our fears, whether to a husband or another godly woman, they are brought into the bright, searing light of God's truth. And when subjected to that light, the fears cannot remain. That's because the very flimsy foundation of fear is believing a lie about who God is—that maybe He doesn't love us or have our best interest in mind, that some things are beyond His control, or that He won't enable us to walk through whatever happens, good or bad.

How to Fight Fear

We cannot take a passive approach in the battle with fear. We must *actively* fight against it. That means kicking out worried thoughts the moment they enter our minds, no matter how logical or "natural" it might feel to give in to them. But in order to do this, we must be equipped with the proper tools.

Often when the temptation to fear arises, it is because of circumstances that are outside your control. But as Martin Luther said, "You cannot keep birds from flying over your head, but you can keep them from building a nest in your hair." The temptation to fear will come, but it is what you do with those thoughts that will make all the difference.

For many years, I couldn't understand why fears I thought I had dealt with kept coming back over and over again. What I didn't see at the time was that my "dealing with them" was actually just sweeping them under the rug, so to speak. When fear came, I would try to ignore it or push it to the back of my mind and distract myself with other things. This seemed to work for a little while, at least until an opportunity arose for those fears to emerge from hiding once more. And they were always a little harder to fight than the last time.

I was between my first and second child when this all came to a head, and I knew something had to change. In the span of about three months, four people I knew (or knew of) lost their young children. I was out running errands when I learned of the fourth child who had died. I got into my car and broke down, weeping uncontrollably. The weight of the grief I felt for those who had lost their children was suffocating. And in that moment, God brought me face to face with my deepest fear: the possibility of losing one of my children.

There was no guarantee that I wouldn't be in that situation one day; it was completely out of my control. I was overwhelmed at the very thought of it. Then the Lord put this question to me: *Do you trust Me? Do you trust that I love you and your children more than you can comprehend, and that if I allow one of your children to be taken from you, I am still holding you in My gentle, loving, all-powerful arms?*

David, the warrior king, said, "When I am afraid, I put my trust in you" (Psalm 56:3). I had to choose. Whom was I going to trust—my fears or my God?

Now I knew exactly what I had to do. I had to cast myself, weak and trembling, upon the Lord and allow His transforming grace to flood my life.

I'm still very much a work in progress, but God is so faithful. Every uncertain situation that would play upon my fears as a mother is another opportunity to entrust my children to Him anew. Every time I choose to trust God in these situations strengthens my confidence in His love, power, and sovereignty.

Let's face it, my fears cannot add a single day to my children's lives, but resting in Jesus makes every one of those days—however many there may be—a time of joy.

As you seek the Lord in this area of your life, let me give you some ways that you can deal with fear head-on.

Know God and Love Him

Hannah Whitall Smith wrote, "Comfort and peace never come from anything we know about ourselves, but only and always from what we know about Him." When we truly know God—His character, His love, His promises—all fear is dispelled from our hearts and minds. It's not enough just to know He exists. We can memorize every Bible passage about worry and repeat them to ourselves a hundred times a day. But if we don't know and love God on a deeply personal and intimate level, then memory verses can only do so much. As 1 John 4:18 tells us, "There is no fear in love, but perfect love casts out fear."

Fill Your Mind with Truth

This goes hand in hand with knowing and loving God. One of the best weapons in the battle against fear is filling our minds with truth. In Ephesians 6, where Paul describes the armor of God, the very first item we are instructed to "put on" is the belt of truth (Ephesians 6:14), for God is the author and source of all truth and fear does not come from Him.

After strapping on the armor of God, the well-dressed Christian mom knows that no outfit is complete without her most important accessory: her Bible. Paul's final instruction concerning the armor of God is to take up "the sword of the Spirit, which is the word of God" (Ephesians 6:17). As Hebrews 4:12 says, "For the word of God is living and active, sharper than any two-edged sword, piercing to the division of soul and of spirit, of joints and of marrow, and discerning the thoughts and intentions of the heart." Scripture has the power to root out wrong thinking and banish all the enemy's lies from our minds. We simply must be diligent to search out the truth and apply it. We must continually keep it at the forefront of our minds throughout the day.

One way of doing this is to write out key scriptures and post them around your home, in places where you know you will see them often. Another "sound" approach is to have an audiobook Bible playing during mealtimes and while you're getting ready in the morning or doing various household tasks. These are my favorite ways of keeping Scripture continually in my mind and heart.

Of course, the best way of hiding God's Word in your heart (Psalm 119:11) is to memorize passages of Scripture. Allow the Lord to inscribe His words on the bedrock of your being, and you will then be able to call them to mind anytime, anyplace, in any situation.

Here are a few of my favorite verses to meditate on when fear tries to overtake me:

> *You keep him in perfect peace whose mind is stayed on you, because he trusts in you. Trust in the LORD forever, for the LORD GOD is an everlasting rock. (Isaiah 26:3–4)*

> *In peace I will both lie down and sleep; for you alone, O LORD, make me dwell in safety. (Psalm 4:8)*

> *The LORD is my light and my salvation; whom shall I fear? The LORD is the stronghold of my life; of whom shall I be afraid? (Psalm 27:1)*

> *[The righteous person] is not afraid of bad news; his heart is firm, trusting in the LORD. (Psalm 112:7)*

> *For God has not given us a spirit of fear, but of power and of love and of a sound mind. (2 Timothy 1:7, NKJV)*

Cultivate a Thankful Heart

Oklahoma City pastor and author Sam Storms is quoted as saying, "Joy is not necessarily the absence of suffering; it is the presence of God." No matter how difficult your circumstances may be, there is always something to praise the Lord for. Even if every single thing is, in fact, going wrong in your daily life, you can thank God for His salvation, His love, His mercy, and His enabling grace to walk through any and every situation.

Even in the best of times, we cannot truly depend on our emotions. Feelings are fickle and are affected by so many things, including what we've eaten and how we slept the night before. So during life's most trying times, when your emotions are being tossed about like a rowboat on a raging sea, lean on what you know to be true about God. For when you're feeling unsure of what's true about yourself, you can always know what's true about the living God. Check out Numbers 23:19, Hebrews 6:18, and James 1:17. See? What was true about the Lord in easier, happier times is still true about Him when the going gets rough, because God never changes!

Now read these passages and leap for joy:

The Lord is at hand; do not be anxious about anything, but in everything by prayer and supplication with thanksgiving let your requests be made known to God. And the peace of God, which surpasses all understanding, will guard your hearts and your minds in Christ Jesus. (Philippians 4:4–6)

Rejoice always, pray without ceasing, give thanks in all circumstances; for this is the will of God in Christ Jesus for you. (1 Thessalonians 5:16–18)

Oh give thanks to the Lord, for he is good, for his steadfast love endures forever! (Psalm 107:1)

When you remember who God is and deliberately turn your heart to Him in gratitude, it will take our eyes off yourself and your problems and onto His glory. You cultivate a thankful heart by calling to mind every day His love and mercy and His promise to see you through any storm:

> *For I, the* Lord *your God, hold your right*
> *hand; it is I who say to you, "Fear not, I am*
> *the one who helps you." (Isaiah 41:13)*

Practice thanking Him every day in every situation, and you will soon be enabled to see beyond your immediate circumstances, knowing that God is in control of every aspect of your life, even if you can't understand what is happening right now.

It was A. W. Tozer who said, "Gratitude is an offering precious in the sight of God, and it is one that the poorest of us can make and not be poorer but richer for having made it."

The Battle Is the Lord's

Second Chronicles 20 tells of a vast military alliance that declared war on good King Jehoshaphat and the nation of Judah. The king himself was terrified by this news, so he called God's people to begin fasting immediately. Then he stood in front the temple in Jerusalem, with the people gathered before him, and he openly prayed for guidance from above.

First, Jehoshaphat confessed his fear, then he acknowledged the power and might of the Lord God and reminded Him how the Lord had delivered the Hebrews from their enemies in times past. Then the king admitted his own powerlessness and that of his people and begged the Lord to help them once more.

Then the Spirit of the Lord came upon one of the men standing there, and the man called out, "This is what the Lord says: Do not be afraid! Don't be discouraged by this mighty army, for the battle is not yours, but God's. ... Do not be afraid or discouraged. Go out against them tomorrow, for the Lord is with you!" (2 Chronicles 20:15–17).

Before my second child was born, I wondered if the worry and fear I had been battling would be doubled with the coming delivery. I confessed my fears to the Lord, praised Him for being my refuge and my shield, and thanked Him for the faithfulness He had shown me time and again. To my amazement, my experience the second time around was exactly opposite from the first. In fact, my joy in motherhood has increased exponentially with each child, and God has given me even more grace to stand against all the "what-ifs" that try to assail me.

To my delight, I have watched the Lord do miracles in my life, beginning the work of transforming me from a fearful, fretting mother-to-be to one who rejoices at the birth to come (Proverbs 31:25). And if He can do that in my life, He will certainly do it in yours as you surrender this area to Him.

Testimony from a Faith-Filled Mama

BROOKE
Mother of Two

On July 1, 2012, I was twenty-five weeks and two days pregnant with our first child. Our sweet boy was nestled safely inside of me, though he was given to occasional outbursts of dancing and boxing. That evening, however, I started having intense back pains that grew steadily worse. Since I had never been in labor before, I didn't know that what I was feeling were contractions. Then my water broke, and we knew we had to dial 9-1-1.

That day, at 9:30 pm, my son came into this world just two pounds, two ounces, via emergency C-section. My scar is a tangible reminder. A mark of love, a story of faith.

And just like that, I was thrust into motherhood. It wasn't quite how I dreamed or how I expected my first days of motherhood to be, and yet the Lord was faithful. And I was given the honor of holding a miracle in my arms and watching him grow every day.

I remember waking from the anesthesia and Josh, my husband, telling me, "We have a son. Josiah Daniel." The nurse wheeled in the Isolette carrying my son, and I placed my finger in his tiny hand. He held it tightly. Then before I knew it, they were whisking him off in a helicopter to another hospital.

That was only the beginning of the journey. We learned trust, faith, and dependence upon the Lord with every wave that threatened to crash upon us during the 114 days our son spent in the hospital. All the while, Jesus was right there beside us, calming us in the midst of the storms. Storms such as four surgeries and watching our son learn how to fill his lungs with oxygen. There were so many mountains to climb, miraculous moments, and opportunities to succumb to fear and worry. In the face of it all, we knew that the Master Artist was weaving our son's story in His perfect wisdom, which extends far beyond our human sight.

Yes, there were times when fear came knocking at the door of my heart, wanting to pull me away, to grasp tightly to the things I love rather than open my hands wide to the Creator and Sustainer of **all** life. But I have learned what it means to trust the Lord wholeheartedly and without abandon. Dealing with our fears doesn't mean pushing away fear and not thinking about it; it's looking fear straight in the face and choosing to cling unwaveringly to the hem of Jesus' garment. I'm choosing to trust in the promises of God, because He who promised is faithful (Hebrews 10:23).

The apostle Peter spoke of "casting all your care upon him, for He cares for you" (1 Peter 5:7, NKJV). The Greek word from which **casting** is derived means to throw off, set down, or cast away from you. In other words, get rid of it! Set down your cares, throw off your anxieties, and give your fears to Almighty God, who called the vast heavens into existence by His mere word. Give your cares to Him, and He will replace your fear with trust, your worry with praise, your anxiety with peace. When in our human frailty we worry that we can't do it or can't handle it, He can. As the saying goes, let go and let God.

Proverbs 31:21–25 shows us a woman who fears the Lord and is not afraid of snow—i.e., hardships and calamity—for her household is clothed in scarlet, and she makes her own bedspreads to keep them warm. She smiles at the future. You and I can smile at the future because we know that we and our dear ones are covered in the finest scarlet: the precious blood of Jesus Christ.

The verse that perhaps best encapsulates our journey from the moment I went into labor with Josiah, to when I had fears of another premature delivery with my second son, David, is Philippians 4:5–7 which says, "The Lord is **at hand**. Be anxious for nothing, but in everything by prayer and supplication, with thanksgiving, let your requests be made known to God; and the **peace** of God, which surpasses **all understanding**, will **guard** your **hearts** and **minds** through Christ Jesus" (NKJV, **italics mine**).

The peace and comfort that come with knowing that He who has held the stars together through the ages is the One who holds all of us. He holds us in the palm of His hand. That is comfort. That is peace that guards a heart and mind. **Cling** to Him, dear sister. Cling to His promises. Cling to the hem of His garment.

We don't have to succumb to the fiery darts the enemy sends our way. No, we can rise up as fearless, valorous women of God and hold up "the shield of faith" to resist the enemy's blows (Ephesians 6:16). As a result, our lives will be so much richer, our faith so much stronger, and the joy of resting on His promises felt ever more deeply.

Motherhood is a treasure, a grand gift the Lord has bestowed on us. It's a tapestry of grace that is woven in the hard moments and the easy moments, the ordinary moments and the extraordinary moments, but each moment, each thread, is a gift.

'Tis so sweet to trust in Jesus.

Choose to trust in Him, my friend.

He will never fail you nor forsake you.

6

PREGNANCY AND HEALTH

For you were bought with a price. So glorify God in your body.
1 Corinthians 6:20

There were plenty of things I enjoyed about prenatal appointments during my first pregnancy. My doctor was kind and attentive, the nurses were fun to interact with, and hearing my baby's heartbeat was always thrilling. But there was one aspect I *never* enjoyed: stepping on the scale. How I dreaded seeing that number moving steadily upward as the weeks went by!

Sometimes my eyes would widen with horror at how much I had gained in such a short time. I was sticking to a healthy diet and staying as active as possible, yet still my weight zoomed past what I thought was reasonable and into a range I had never before seen associated with my own body.

After each appointment I found myself praying, asking the Lord to help me win the battle for my mind. I asked Him to remind me that my worth is found in Him, not in how much I weigh, and that it was a privilege to carry this little life inside me, no matter what happened to my body in the process.

During my early teen years, I had begun to struggle with my appearance. I was extremely self-conscious most of the time. I had many friends who were petite, and although I wasn't very big, I definitely was not little. I lived in an Asian country where most of the clothing that fit me was labeled "XXL." I would often catch myself comparing aspects of my appearance to those around me, and as the years went by, my concerns over my weight became an obsession—a stronghold that walled off more and more of my heart and mind. I was miserable so much of the time that, many mornings, I didn't even want try to pick out clothing and get dressed for the day.

I was also walking through some health struggles that caused my weight to fluctuate quite a bit, regardless of what I ate. I actually maintained a pretty healthy diet and exercised almost every day, but my body seemed to have a mind of its own in regard to gaining or losing weight. Meanwhile, my emotions went up and down with the number on the scale. I was able to put on a happy, carefree demeanor most of the time, but inside I was in turmoil.

I knew this wasn't right thinking, but I had no idea how to change my thoughts. I wanted so badly to be free from the snare of insecurity and self-focus. Desperate, I finally cried out to the Lord for help. And although it wasn't an overnight transformation, He began the process of bringing me out of bondage. I longed for the glorious freedom to fix my eyes on Him rather than keeping my gaze fixed upon myself and my weight.

Pregnancy proved to be the turning point for me in surrendering this area of my life to Jesus. He used my pregnancies to show me that my body was for more than keeping in shape or being attractive for my husband. This body was being used to grow a new life! And in order for that life to thrive, I had to be physically grown, stretched, and changed in my appearance. I had to give up my obsession with looking a certain way and be okay with that number on the scale (rapidly) rising. But the Lord wasn't just asking me to be flexible regarding my weight; He was retraining my mind to think from His perspective.

In this chapter, we're going to focus on three things: eating, exercise, and sleep. These can be touchy topics for women, especially during pregnancy. The message we often hear when expecting is that it's perfectly normal for a mom-to-be to give in to self-indulgence, eating whatever she craves and sleeping her days away. Then there are those who, as I did, go to the opposite extreme and obsess about every ounce they gain, even resenting the fact that their body is changing and doing all they can to hold on to their pre-pregnancy figure. Neither of these is based in right thinking. Of course, when you're pregnant, your calorie intake *needs* to be higher, and you *do* need rest more often. But even these are to be harnessed by God's Spirit and used for His glory, just as when we are not pregnant.

In 1 Corinthians 10:31, Paul says, "So, whether you eat or drink, or whatever you do, do all to the glory of God." He doesn't say, "Except when you are pregnant; then you can do whatever you want!" In 1 Corinthians 6:19–20, he says, "Or do you not know that your body is a temple of the Holy Spirit within you, whom you have from God? You are not your own, for you were bought with a price. So glorify God in your body." Anyone who is indwelled by the Holy Spirit falls into this category. As Christians, we are to glorify God *all the time*. If we make excuses or ease up on self-control because it's harder during pregnancy, we are treading on dangerous ground. Think of all the examples from Paul's life. Imprisonment, shipwrecks, multiple beatings, stoning, persecution—the list goes on and on. (Read the full account in 2 Corinthians 11:24–33). How did he respond to these hardships?

> *But [the Lord] said to me, "My grace is sufficient for you, for my power is made perfect in weakness." Therefore, I will boast all the more gladly of my weaknesses, so that*

the power of Christ may rest upon me. For the sake of Christ, then, I am content with weaknesses, insults, hardships, persecutions, and calamities. For when I am weak, then I am strong. (2 Corinthians 12:9–10)

It is when we are at our weakest that God's power can be most wonderfully and beautifully displayed, giving us the grace to love when we don't want to, serve when we feel we have nothing left to give, choose joy in the midst of our difficulties, and in this case, practice self-control when our cravings are strongest. This is not a legalistic thing or something we need to be paranoid about. It is simply having the heart determination that says, *Lord, I want to honor you with every part of my life, and that includes taking care of my body during this season when my motivation sometimes waver. But I know your grace is available to me all the time!*

Eating

I had been on a pretty strict diet for several months prior to becoming pregnant with my first child. I had been dealing with some digestive issues and trying to get into shape. But I realized fairly quickly that I needed to rethink my eating habits while I was expecting. This meant adding back to my diet certain foods I had been avoiding—grains, fruits, and certain vegetables—so that I wasn't depriving my baby and my body of nutrients we would need for the next nine months. I was surprised to find that in reintroducing these foods I had been avoiding, my body actually thrived to the point that many of my previous digestive issues were almost nonexistent!

As I sought to walk in wisdom, God supplied it. I seemed to know instinctually which foods were good for me and which foods weren't ideal for my pregnant body. I knew when it was okay to have a little treat and when I should abstain. God used that season to teach me a lot about how to be wise and discerning with my food choices.

For a long time, I had been downright legalistic about my sugar intake. Of course, we all know that consuming too much sugar isn't good for us. Practicing self-control in this area is always a good idea, but I had become paranoid about accidentally consuming foods that contained even a trace of sugar. While everyone else was enjoying the church potluck, I was worrying about my weight and frantically trying to figure out how I was going to fit in another hour of exercise that week. Now, the desire to be healthy is a good thing, but my motivations and priorities were wrongheaded. I was focused on myself and my appearance and making lifestyle choices based on my insecurities. It was incredibly freeing when I was able to let go of this mindset and allow the Lord to reshape my thinking about food.

I still strive to be a good steward of my body. It is the temple of the Holy Spirit, after all. But I am no longer in bondage to the food I eat or don't eat. Rather than stressing about every calorie or giving in to every craving that comes along, I simply choose to walk daily in a way that is honoring to the Lord.

If you find yourself on one side or the other, either too concerned about what you're putting into your body or not practicing enough self-control, it is important to give God control of this area of your life. Seek Him for wisdom in making eating choices that are healthy for both you and for the little one inside your womb.

Sometimes it's tricky to know how to do this. Some choices are black-and-white, leaving no doubt whether we should or should not consume certain things when we're pregnant. For instance, we know that consuming alcoholic beverages can have terrible consequences for the developing child, so that's a big NO for Mama.[1] We also know that caffeine is a stimulant that can keep us from getting a good night's sleep—the jury is still out on other, more serious side effects—so Mama needs to be careful with her caffeine intake.[2]

But other food and beverage choices aren't so clear-cut. How much sugar is okay to eat? What if even the thought of a vegetable makes you want to lose your lunch? What if all you can stomach for lunch are gluten-free shortbread cookies? Cravings and aversions are difficult to navigate during pregnancy, and God knows this. Don't hesitate to go to Him for wisdom. Nothing is too small to bring before the Lord.

It glorifies God when you choose to involve Him in whatever you are walking through. Here are some ways to begin bringing your dietary choices in line with His will for you.

Ask God for Wisdom

One of my favorite Bible verses says, "If any of you lacks wisdom, let him ask of God who gives generously to all without reproach, and it will be given him" (James 1:5). I have experienced the truth of this statement more times than I can count! It's true all day, every day, even between meals. If you're quick to snack on anything that looks good without giving it a second thought, ask God for wisdom to know when you should practice more self-control. If you are tempted to eat less than you know you should because the idea of gaining weight makes your stomach churn, ask God to give you wisdom to know what is best for you and your child and what will glorify Him. Believe me, the wisdom will be there right when you need it.

Eating in Moderation

As a rule of thumb, moderation is a good place to start when choosing what to eat. This is especially true when talking about certain foods that aren't *terrible* for you or the baby but probably aren't the best choice either.

What "moderation" really boils down to is self-control. Merriam-Webster's definition of *self-control* is "restraint exercised over one's own impulses, emotions, or desires." Self-control is not simply saying no to everything; it's knowing the right amount of something to have and sticking to that. Too much of anything, even good things, can end up being . . . well, not so good. Eating one Hershey's Kiss won't kill you. Drinking one cup of coffee probably isn't going to do you any harm. But if you find that you can't stop at one or two pieces of chocolate, or you're running back to the Keurig all day for another pick-me-up, you may need to consider cutting these things out altogether for a while.

Generally, self-control is a matter of knowing how much of a food is the right amount for you. The "right amount" will vary from woman to woman, and each of us is responsible to make those decisions in a Christ-honoring manner. Consider making a list of foods and beverages you enjoy that offer few required nutrients. Ask yourself, *Am I practicing self-control when it comes to these things? Which of these do I have a hard time eating or drinking in moderation?*

Some of my friends choose to avoid all caffeine during their pregnancy, and others don't. Some of my friends eliminate all sugar during pregnancy, and others don't. But in each of their lives I see a pattern of self-control and a desire to honor the Lord and do what is best for her baby.

Getting Creative

During the early weeks of my second pregnancy, I found that water was one of the culprits triggering my bouts of morning sickness. Obviously, this was a problem, and it didn't take long before I became dehydrated. So I tried drinking carbonated water—a.k.a. soda water, sparkling water, or seltzer—which worked *much* better. This allowed me to stay hydrated without having to rely on sugary drinks. Then there was the time when the only thing edible that sounded good was gluten-free shortbread cookies, which I knew I couldn't live off of for very long without courting disaster. But after trying a few things, I discovered that bananas were a good alternative that helped my digestion and provided vitamin B6 for my baby.

Even after morning sickness fades, there are times when those cravings hit hard, and it's all a pregnant mom can do to keep from consuming an entire container of ice cream in one sitting. But again, if you ask, God will give you the wisdom to know when a serving or two of ice cream is okay and when it's better to look elsewhere to satisfy your needs. Maybe instead of ice cream, try some plain Greek yogurt sweetened with maple syrup and blueberries. Or perhaps a piece of dark chocolate instead of a Snickers bar. Remember, this has nothing to do with legalism but has everything to do with wisdom—understanding what is best for the baby, and best for you, in the long run.

Exercise

Personally, I really enjoy exercise—most of the time. Even so, like most people, I need to be motivated to start and continue a steady habit of exercise. And my resistance is taken to a whole other level when morning sickness is in full swing and pregnancy fatigue has me dragging my feet all day. As the months wear on, there's back pain and nerve pain and ... well, you get the idea.

Due to issues like iron deficiency, dehydration, and severe sciatica at various times in my pregnancies, I found it difficult to stay consistent in this area, and there were times when it wasn't wise for me to even try. But the desire to honor God and provide the best for my baby was helpful motivation to make healthy choices even when I couldn't be very active.

In fitness as in life, our daily choices should ultimately be guided by love. Jesus says our top priority at all times is to love God with all that we have and are (Luke 10:27), and I figure this probably means performing at least basic maintenance on the body He's entrusted to my care. Then there's the little person we are carrying around inside when pregnant. For some of us, making the loving choice might mean choosing to exercise even when it's the last thing we want to do. For others, it may mean choosing to rest rather than exerting energy we don't have just to maintain a desirable body weight.

After love comes wisdom. The choices we make with our body, such as whether to exercise or not, will have consequences that are either good or bad. If I am not exercising yet giving into every craving I have, what will be the result once I don't have the excuse of being pregnant? I'm not talking about having the same body you had before pregnancy. I completely understand, from experience, that a woman's body goes through drastic changes during pregnancy and for months afterward. Some women, no matter how hard they try, cannot seem to take the extra weight off and will never fit back into a size six. But if, during pregnancy, they were striving to do what was best for the baby and their own health while glorifying the Lord, then that is all that matters.

Here are a few tips that may help you to make healthy choices regarding exercise while carrying your child.

Start Small and Be Consistent
You don't have to spend an hour at the gym every day to stay active during pregnancy. Regular exercise can mean a daily walk around the neighborhood or climbing the staircase at home a couple of extra times. If you have other children, exercise can be throwing a ball back and forth, pulling weeds together, or having a dance party with them (if they're anything like mine). Maybe it's going to the pool, walking the dog, or choosing to park your car a little farther away at the store just to get a few more steps in. Be creative and find ways to make it fun!

Enroll in a Class
During my second pregnancy, I enrolled in a Pilates class. I told the instructor beforehand that I was expecting, and she tailored

my exercises to be safe for me. The class provided great motivation and helped me to retain more flexibility while warding off back and nerve pain a little bit longer. Consider looking into exercise classes in your area that are pregnancy-friendly. If you're able, go for it!

Seriously, Don't Stress About It

Stress has the potential to counteract your best efforts to take care of your body. Stressed-out moms sleep poorly, exercise less, and tend to fall back into unhealthy eating patterns. If you are constantly fretting about staying in shape, getting every step in, and worrying about every pound, your concerns are taking away from the joy of pregnancy. Exercise should be a means of *reducing* worry and stress, not contributing to them. So if you are struggling with being too concerned, take it before the Lord and ask Him to help you develop the right perspective. Ask Him for help to be joyful and thankful for this new and exciting season and for the grace to accept each change as it comes.

Sleep

Everyone who's been with child knows that pregnancy fatigue is no joke. I could not believe how utterly wiped out I felt for the nine months leading up to the birth of my first child. I would wake up at 8:00 every morning and, after eating and getting ready for the day, be ready for a nap by 9:00. By the time 7:00 p.m. rolled around, I was exhausted and ready to crawl into bed—then repeat the whole cycle the next day!

While it's true that a woman's body needs considerably more rest in this season of life, the temptation to *over*indulge in sleep can be strong. It's hard to find the right balance, as we tend toward one extreme or the other: giving in to the urge to sleep too much, depriving our bodies of the rest they need by staying up too late, overcommitting ourselves, trying to maintain appearances, and so on. Sometimes I find myself tempted toward both extremes. There are certain days I want to give in to laziness, particularly when my schedule calls for doing a task I don't really enjoy; other days I neglect my need for rest because I have simply taken on too many things. It's a balancing act that requires wisdom only the Lord can provide, for only He fully understands our individual needs and unique circumstances. One person may need to set aside a few planned tasks to get some much-needed rest, while another person might need to push through the fatigue a little longer. And God will give grace for both (2 Corinthians 12:9).

During each of my pregnancies, there were a few helpful questions I asked myself when trying to decide if I should lie down for a quick nap. These have helped me to understand whether my motives were right and in keeping with godly principles.

Are There Urgent Tasks to Complete?

Yes, sometimes that load of laundry can wait. Or those dishes can be done later. But sometimes there are tasks I *know* I need to complete before taking a nap; otherwise, I will be setting myself up for greater exhaustion and/or anxiety a few hours from now. Many times, if I'm efficient about completing the task, I will still have a little time to rest (and this time with a quieted mind). Thinking this way can help a mom to get the work done and lessens the urge to procrastinate.

Before I move on to the next question, you've probably heard it said before, but it is *so* true: If you have young children, the best way to fit in a nap is during the kids' nap time. Planning to lay down when your kids do is helpful motivation to complete the tasks that need doing, knowing there will be a structured and predictable time for rest.

Do I Need to Set Aside Technology for a Time?

While you're resting, resist the urge to turn to technology every time. I know from personal experience that this is a hard one, but it's an absolute necessity. It's all too easy—again, speaking from experience—to lie down for a nap or bedtime at night and get distracted by technology. Not only does checking social media in bed keep us from going to sleep, but using our screens late in the evening has been shown to lower the quality of sleep we're getting once we *do* put our phones and tablets away.

I always find that I'm far more refreshed, both mentally and physically, when I keep my phone and computer turned off during my times of rest. Also, I have found it helpful to set boundaries for myself as to when to put away my gadgets for the night and at what point I can pick them up in the morning. Ask the Lord to show you if technology is hindering you from getting the rest you need and, if so, guide you as to what changes you need to make in this area.

One last thought about keeping technology in proper perspective: When I choose to set aside my phone and play with my kiddos, I am freed from the tyranny of the phone and allowed to cherish my children without distraction. Being with them fully in body *and* mind has created some precious moments I will always treasure.

Am I Finding My Rest in the One Who Is Rest?

I cannot emphasize enough the importance of making time with Jesus a priority. It is only in Him that true rest is found. I am the kind of person who can get a little panicky when I'm functioning on too little sleep. And sadly, I have too often skipped my quiet time with the Lord to get a little extra physical rest, even though I know I'm missing out on something *far* more important than even sleep. I can't tell you what a difference it makes in my day if I have set aside time to focus on Him that morning. When

I choose to climb out of bed in the morning and find my rest in Jesus, I find I'm not nearly as stressed about missing sleep or getting all my to-do list done. He promises in Matthew 11:28, "Come to me, all who labor and are heavy laden, and I will give you rest."

Hannah Whitall Smith put it this way: "No soul can really be at rest until it has given up all dependence on everything else and has been forced to depend on the Lord alone. As long as our expectation is from other things, nothing but disappointment awaits us."[3]

A Final Word

As a final word, I just want to state again: This is *not* law. Eating habits, exercise, and rest will look different for each woman in pregnancy, and their proper use requires daily wisdom. We are each responsible to seek the Lord individually to know what will honor Him most. Don't fret about the changes taking place in your body or worry about a number on the scale—those things will only steal your joy. Take these things to Jesus, knowing that He has given you this child to carry. What a privilege! So rejoice in the Lord and dedicate these areas of your life to Him.

Testimony from a Wise Mama

SHELLY
Mother of Eight

I recently gave birth to our eighth child, and let's just say I am not on the younger side of the spectrum when it comes to having babies. Now that it's over, I am grateful for my healthy son, but I'm also thankful for all I have learned through my many pregnancies. For example, I am a much more relaxed mom these days. This is due in part to my realizing how short life is and how much God works things out when we really give our cares to Him.

One of the most important things I have learned through eight pregnancies is that having no plan for exercise, sleep, and eating leads to a rough road ahead. Just having a few general thoughts or fuzzy, big-picture ideas without a detailed plan for following through is a sure recipe for feeling exasperated and overwhelmed at the end of each day. Such feelings are not what God has in mind when He promises in 2 Peter 1:3 that His divine power has given us all things pertaining to life and godliness, which presumably includes what we need for childbearing. But what does that look like practically?

Although I haven't had to endure a high-risk pregnancy or extreme difficulties while expecting, pregnancy nevertheless can be a demanding and challenging time for me. Of course, I don't start my days planning to become overwhelmed. In fact, I usually enjoy a purposeful time with Jesus each morning in preparation to live out a victorious, joyful day. Why then at the end of my day do I sometimes have those negative feelings? Simply put, the problem is physical fatigue.

While having babies is one of the highest privileges in my life, pregnancy is also physically draining for me, and as we know, fatigue sometimes leads to mental weakness. Thankfully, I know that my weakness is an opportunity for the Lord to work powerfully in my life, so I'm okay with depending on His strength. Sometimes, this means leaning on the gifts He has given me, such as my husband.

I confess that when I 'm tired, I have a harder time thinking clearly and making decisions. So I often turn to my husband for help. I want to make my health a priority, so I will ask him to pray with me to make wise food choices. Sometimes I will ask his help in finding someone to watch the children for an hour or handle a couple of my errands so I can use that time to exercise. Exercise combats stress and brightens my mood.

I find it's a good idea for me to exercise earlier in the day, because it's when I have the most energy, and doing it early means I'm not tempted to skip it later in the day if my to-do list gets backed up. During my last few pregnancies, I walked an hour each morning while listening to sermons. During my most recent pregnancy, I participated in a water exercise class that really helped my joints and greatly reduced the back pain I experienced in previous pregnancies. But in order to make time for morning walks and swim classes, I had to alter my usual morning routine, and it helped tremendously to talk this through with my husband and get his feedback.

Rest and sleep are vital for recharging my body each day. This may mean going to bed pretty early to make time for morning exercise. "Pretty early" can mean 8 p.m., and sometimes the house isn't quite as organized or clean as I'd like by that hour. I ask the children to help the best they can, but some chores can only be done by me or the older children, so that may mean being okay with leaving a chore or two until the next day. I'm happy to report that they get done somehow by the grace of God!

Rest also means simplifying my schedule so that my days move at a somewhat slower pace. When I'm not pregnant, I'm perfectly capable of managing multiple household tasks and outside activities. But trying to maintain that same pace when pregnant takes a real toll on my body, so changes must be made. Rest also helps to lower my stress, which lowers the stress on the baby growing inside of me. I think about that quite a bit when I'm pregnant. The problem isn't so much worry and anxiety; I know those things are bad for me, and we're commanded in God's Word not to do them. Rather, it's about the pace of life I'm keeping. There have been some pregnancies that required me to scale back my activities outside the home almost completely. Other times, I was capable of doing more, and so I did.

Meal preparation during pregnancy is simplified for our family too. I don't love the smells of many foods when pregnant, but I work through it the best I can. I use the crockpot quite a bit during those months so the kids can serve up their own food when I can't seem to move my body late in the day. We generally eat quite healthy as a family, but I've learned that's not a realistic goal every single night when I'm with child.

When my older kids were young, dinner was sometimes fish sticks or sandwiches with a salad. These days I've learned to make use of those times when I have more energy to do extra cooking for the week ahead. And I am amazed how much my children have creatively produced food-wise when asked!

As for my diet, I have a bigger appetite when I'm pregnant, so it's important I fill up on nourishing whole foods, plenty of fruits and vegetables, and whole grains. After my morning walk, I usually make a big fruit-and-protein smoothie or a hearty egg-and-toast breakfast that leaves me full until lunch. I find it's better if I eat regularly and promptly, and that means a nourishing lunch, followed by a midafternoon snack of fruit and nuts or perhaps another smoothie.

These are some tips that have worked well for me over the years, and I hope they will bless you too as you carry your little gift from God.

7

PREGNANCY AND LIFESTYLE

For God is not a God of confusion but of peace.
1 Corinthians 14:33

One frosty evening in December found me holding our third child just hours after she was born. I was exhausted but overjoyed. I chatted with the night shift nurse whenever she came in to take our temperatures or check my blood pressure. Early the next morning as she was getting ready to leave for the day, she said, "You're kind of famous around here." Curious, I asked why. She said, "When you came in late one night a couple of weeks ago to be monitored, I was sitting at the nurse's station with a couple of other nurses. Because of the way you were dressed, we said to each other, 'She's a first-timer for sure!' We were surprised to learn this is actually your third baby. No one comes in looking that nice so late at night when they're expecting their third!"

I remembered the clothing I had on that evening, and it really didn't seem like much—jeans, sweater, and my maternity peacoat. But this wasn't the first time someone had complimented the way I looked during my third trimester. I'd received a handful of similar comments late in both my second and third pregnancies.

In choosing my maternity wardrobe each day, I made decisions based on what I would normally wear. I did my hair the way I would have if I weren't pregnant. I put on my makeup the same way. And yet, ladies like the night-shift nurse always seemed surprised that, even with multiple children and one on the way, I had any semblance of being put together.

Everyone who's ever been pregnant has heard the dire pronouncements:

"Having a baby will change everything, and sometimes not for the better."

"You will never sleep again."

"Your house will be a disaster and the atmosphere chaotic."

"You *might* get to shower every five days."

"You will live in yoga pants."

"You'll be lucky each day if you're able to swipe on some mascara and throw your hair into a haphazard ponytail before running out the door."

"You will feel harried and frazzled and overwhelmed pretty much all the time. But you'll survive. Just remember—chaos can be beautiful!"

"Even a mom who is pure in heart and says her prayers by night may become a monster when the wolfbane blooms and nap time is over."

Okay, maybe that last one is a bit extreme. But I can't tell you how many "mom blogs" and movies and talk shows and even Christian women I've known share such ominous warnings as though they're dispensing *helpful* advice. Before your child has left the womb, you will likely have been prepared for the "perils" that lie ahead by more than one well-meaning mom. As a result, maybe you're already approaching your due date with a sense of discouragement, foreboding, and even hopelessness.

But do such prophecies of doom have to be true? Is that really how God intends motherhood to be? Is pregnancy just a time to steel ourselves against the dark days to come?

I don't think so.

Our God Is a God of Order

When God created the world, He did it in an orderly way. Scientists always seem to be discovering very specific, intricate systems that keep this world working, and working well. God didn't just "wing it." He designed every aspect of His creation to reflect beauty and order. When God had Solomon and the Israelites build the first temple in Jerusalem, it was done in a very systematic and coherent way, so that it reverberated with facets of God's character. Everything in the house of the Lord was to be "done decently and in order" (1 Corinthians 14:40).

The tenor of our lives should be in accordance with this as well. If we have been born again, indwelled with the life of Christ, and are being sanctified by His Spirit, then our internal reality should be one of beauty, order, and peace. We are to be steady, joyful, and life-giving as an overflow of the life and love at work within us. This order and peace should also be manifested in the way we run our homes and present ourselves.

Proverbs 31 paints a picture of the ultimate example of godly femininity. In this chapter we find descriptions like these:

Her clothing is fine linen and purple. (v. 22)

Strength and dignity are her clothing, and she laughs at the time to come. (v.25)

She looks well to the ways of her household and does not eat the bread of idleness. (v. 27)

*Her children rise up and call her blessed; her
husband also, and he praises her. (v. 28)*

This is a woman who does not let chaos reign in her home.
She isn't constantly disheveled and frazzled. She doesn't let anxiety
cloud her actions or attitude. She is strong, diligent, resourceful,
hard-working, and joyful.

Is this an impossible standard to live up to in your own
strength? Absolutely! But *in God's strength*, it is something He
delights to create in you when you depend completely upon Him.

My friend Leslie Ludy has written about motherhood:

> *Exchanging chaos for order and peace may feel like an
> impossible task. But the good news is that it's not a task
> we need to accomplish in our own strength or willpower.
> God Himself is interested in the details of our home and
> family life. He alone can equip us to build our households
> into a reflection of His orderly, peaceful nature.*
>
> *Remember, embracing God's pattern for order doesn't
> mean we'll never experience chaos. Rather, it means that
> we know that God has more for us, and therefore we
> refuse to accept chaos as the end result of our mothering.[1]*

This is my desire—to have the order, peace, and beauty of
Jesus be reflected in my appearance and in the way I keep my
home. These are the spheres where I have the most immediate
influence, and it's important that I care for them in a way that
glorifies the Lord.

Legalism vs. Faithfulness

There is a fine line between doing something out of legalism and
doing it faithfully and heartily "as for the Lord" (Colossians 3:23).
The most significant difference is the *attitude* that accompanies
what you do.

Think about this for a moment. You can keep a house that sparkles or be sure your outward appearance is always perfectly polished, but if your motivation in doing these things is to draw attention to yourself, to make people think more highly of you, or to meet some kind of perceived standard you feel you need to live up to, then your efforts are all in vain. If your heart's motivation in anything is to bring glory to yourself rather than giving glory to God, then your misguided efforts will leave you empty, stressed, exhausted, unfulfilled, and distanced from your family and friends.

Please don't misunderstand. Working to maintain your household and taking a little bit of care to be presentable are *good things.* Just because you might have the wrong motives doesn't mean you should throw out *what* you are doing, but it does mean you need to ask the Lord to help you adjust your thinking regarding *why* and *how* you do it. You can keep a similar cleaning schedule and wear many of the same clothes, yet do so with a heart to glorify God, love and serve your family, and respect the people who visit your home or come into contact with you.

If you will put God and His glory first in everything you do, you will find that you're no longer frazzled and worn at the end of each day. Instead, you will find that you go to bed filled with joy, knowing you have done everything for Him. Will you still be physically tired? Probably. Defeated and discouraged? No.

It's All About the Heart

Now, before I go into the "practicals" of a lifestyle that honors and glorifies the Lord, I need to emphasize again that this is *not* about having a perfect home or appearance. Goodness, I would be treading dangerously near the height of hypocrisy if that's the message I were proclaiming! If you could be a fly on the wall in my home on a regular day, you'd see that it is rarely in pristine shape and that sometimes I'm in my PJs until noon.

I am definitely a work-in-progress. (Some days I feel like an entire construction zone!) But I am learning to nurture a heart for honoring the Lord with my home and my outward appearance. To that end, I am continually seeking Him in how to best do these things. I believe our homes and appearance should be a reflection of the internal peace and joy that comes from being transformed by Jesus. But that peace won't be evident in the external parts of my life unless His peace is first internalized. Even in the moments when there are Cheerios all over the freshly swept floor or I discover food remnants stuck to my growing belly—yes, true story—I know my home can still be filled with joy and calm if I choose to realize that I am not a victim to chaos but, rather, a cultivator of good.

Our Homes

Jani Ortlund has written, "I believe that a godly home is a foretaste of heaven. Our homes, imperfect as they are, must be a haven from the chaos outside. They should be a reflection of our eternal home, where troubled souls find peace, weary hearts find rest, hungry bodies find refreshment, lonely pilgrims find communion, and wounded spirits find compassion."[2] Jani's words capture the heart I have for my home. This is a vision I learned from my mom, who learned it from *her* mom. I have watched both of them make their homes into places that reflect Christ's peace and joy, even when children are filling every room.

I can't tell you how many times I heard people say after visiting my parents' home, "Your home is so peaceful! I love being there! Are you sure there were eight kids in here?" The funny thing is, there were usually more like twelve or fourteen kids in our house at any one time in the afternoons. Our home was a place where everyone wanted to be. It wasn't always perfectly clean, but there was usually a sense of order and a spirit of joy. There weren't always gourmet meals on the stove, but love went into making every tuna melt and stir-fry.

What contributed to this atmosphere of order and joy more than anything was that both my parents were committed to building a home that glorified God. At their wedding, they sang a song together called "Household of Faith." It's a Steve Green song, and its lyrics speak of loving one another unselfishly and making the home "a place that fully abounds with grace" as a reflection of God's face.

I saw this lived out every single day. Before anyone came for dinner, my dad would say, "We are going to be a blessing to those who are coming into our home." This mindset was instilled in us, and its massive impact on me is one I am still only beginning to realize. It was my parents' determination to reflect Christ that made our house a place of rest and refreshment for all who entered there.

Despite the many social changes since we were children, the condition of our homes should still reflect this principle: *God will be glorified in our home, and we commit to doing whatever must be done to make this a reality.*

When a husband and wife take this principle to heart, living it out and teaching it to their children, it overflows into every area of the home—cleaning, cooking, decorating, parenting, hospitality, which movies we choose to watch or not watch, and so on. Of course, the more you try to keep this principle, the more you will see that it's impossible to do in your own strength. This will keep you and your family going back to the Lord again and again, knowing that time spent in His presence, hiding His Word in your heart, and communing with Him in prayer are the only things that will ultimately hold that commitment together.

Every single morning, my mother was up before the sun. I was often the first child up, especially as a teenager, so I would occasionally catch a glimpse of my mom's morning times with the Lord. I would go to the living room to see the soft glow of candles and my mom kneeling by our sofa and reading the Bible, journaling, or praying. She knew that in order to raise her eight children, be a loving wife, pour herself out for others, and keep her home, she *needed* that time in His presence.

She still does it faithfully to this day, although most of her children are now grown. I have seen her plow through a day on very little sleep, making meals for twenty-plus people, doing three or four loads of laundry, praying with someone who calls her in need of encouragement, chatting with a person who stops in unexpectedly, taking hours to talk with a child who is struggling, yet making sure the kitchen is clean before she goes to bed. And do you know what? Her attitude is one of consistent peace and joy, even when she is totally drained physically. My mom never complains. In fact, she usually is thinking about other ways she wishes she could have helped someone. This is not something that comes from her own strength but from years and years of faithfully seeking the Lord and knowing that her strength comes from Him.

With Children Comes ... Mess

I've often fallen into the trap of thinking that the standard for being a good keeper of my home is the absence of messes (which makes me feel like a failure every day that's not the case). But my mother-in-law reminded me of this verse a few years ago in the context of a caring for a home, and it was incredibly encouraging: "Where there are no oxen, the manger is clean, but abundant crops come by the strength of the ox" (Proverbs 14:4). She was basically making the point that where there are children, there is going to be a mess; yet children are a blessing, and ultimately, it is a strength to have them (Psalm 127:3–5).

It's simply not possible to keep everything in a home perfectly clean at every point in the day. And during pregnancy, when morning sickness makes it nearly impossible to clean the dishes and back pain sometimes keeps you from getting the bathrooms clean, it's *okay* if things don't look perfect. I have to remind myself of this often. Yes, I am called to do my best with what has been given to me, but if my current calling—in this case, pregnancy—is preventing me from keeping on top of every little mess, then I can rest in God's grace, knowing that our spiritual lives matter most.

Keeping your home can either be a great burden or a great joy. When your focus turns away from Christ and onto all the things that need to get done—especially any unexpected tasks that arise or extra messes your children make—then it's easy to become discouraged, frustrated, and depressed. But when you continue to fix your eyes on Jesus, keeping your sights on the eternal value of each thing He puts in front of you, it's possible to survive even the most trying of days and emerge on the other side with a heartful of praise and peace in Him.

When you're anticipating a little one—or *another* little one—it's tempting to fixate on all the things that will change and wonder how in the world you'll be able to handle all the feedings and changings and unexpected diaper blowouts, especially if this little one insists on doing these things after everyone else has gone to bed. Just the thought of these added responsibilities can become overwhelming and stressful before the child is even born.

But, sweet mother, don't you fear. This season of pregnancy is the perfect time to begin putting things into practice that will help you turn your home into a haven of rest for every person who enters, even if a few toys are scattered about the floor or there are dirty dishes in the sink. Here are a few simple, practical tips that I have found to be so helpful in maintaining a household before and after this season of preparation.

A Little Planning Goes a Long Way

I love keeping a regular schedule, but I have a difficult time putting one together when I begin thinking of all the things that need to be done. I tend to get overwhelmed by the big picture rather than just choosing a task or two and getting them done. Thankfully, I have a husband who is excellent at helping me break down the big picture into a reasonable and totally doable to-do list. I highly suggest this approach as a place to start.

First, write down each task that needs to get done, then prioritize these from most important to least important. Next, choose two or three of the top-priority tasks to do today and save the rest for tomorrow or the next day. If you put ten tasks on your list but only get five of them accomplished, you'll no doubt be discouraged that you accomplished only half the items on your list. If, however, you put three tasks on your list and accomplish five, you will feel super-productive. Let me tell you, it's a wonderful feeling!

My husband and I use a task organization program and app called Todoist. It has been so helpful in keeping track of everything that needs to get done, especially when I'm in the midst of "pregnancy brain," which comes back full force for me with every pregnancy. I also highly recommend reading Tim Challies's book *Do More Better: A Practical Guide to Productivity*, which walks you through several practical tools for managing your time and information. The book is short and simple and has been a tremendous help to me as a homemaker and mother!

Alternate Your Tasks and Rest

I know what it's like to want to lay around all day because my energy level is at an all-time low and pregnancy symptoms are at an all-time high. I've found that keeping a task/rest mentality always helps. For example, I clean the bathroom and then rest for twenty minutes. I do the dishes, then rest for another twenty minutes. This way, I am getting things accomplished without exhausting my energy reserves, and I am motivated by the reward of getting a little more rest at the end of each task.

We moms need to be balanced in our approach toward work and rest. Some people think of rest (outside of sleeping at night) as a negative thing; they see it as laziness. But rest is a good and needed thing, as God knew when He instituted the Sabbath for His people. In fact, we are also commanded to set apart times for just being still in His presence (Psalm 46:10). It's easy to dismiss sitting and being quiet as a poor use of our time, but if we're using that time to focus on the Lord and meditate on His Word, then it's incredibly good for us.

As you're preparing to be a mom (or adding another child to the family), setting aside regular times to think and pray throughout your day proves to be so helpful, even vital, in preparing mentally for the changes to come. The Lord has used many of my quiet moments to bring to light a fear I'd been harboring, a new idea for handling a parenting struggle, or something I needed to talk with my husband about concerning the coming baby.

I love Psalm 143:5, which reads, "I remember the days of old; I meditate on all that you have done; I ponder the work of your hands." Putting the mind to "work" by thinking about the things of God and those things that glorify Him is actually a form of deep rest for us. In my experience, this is *far* more restful than browsing Facebook for an hour. Make it a habit starting now to ponder the things of God several times a day. I believe you'll find that you're more productive in the long run when you make time for Him.

Work as a Team

Chances are your husband has a way of thinking that's different from yours, at least in some ways. Treasure this fact. I can't tell you how many times I've been stumped trying to set up a practical system that addresses a certain need or issue and my husband then offered a brilliant idea on how to make it happen. For instance, we both like to be organized, but this preference manifests itself differently for each of us. I like to group things with like things—e.g., bakeware is stored *only* with other baking items. Judah, on the other hand, loves the challenge of fitting as many things as possible into a space, even if the various items don't necessarily "go together." Wasn't it on Sesame Street that they used to sing, "One of these things is not like the others ... but that's okay as long as it can be made to fit in the space without folding, spindling, or mutilating"?

In our first apartment, we had very limited storage and only a few cabinets in the kitchen. Judah helped me figure out ways to make everything fit in an orderly manner, even if it meant having to store baking supplies with the knives. And it was Judah's technique for folding clothing that helped me to consistently keep my drawers in order, after trying my whole life to do so! The fact that he is a visionary and I am a get-it-done gal makes us a great team. He draws me out of the box I am used to thinking in.

Your husband might not love or even care about setting up organizational systems, but it's always worth seeking his advice and including him in the daily running of the home. He might surprise you with an inventive solution or two that would never have occurred to you. And even if his suggestions don't appeal to you or won't work for some reason, receive his advice with humility and thankfulness. He will be honored that you wanted to include him.

Include Your Children

As of this writing, I have four children under the age of seven. It's easy to fall into the mindset that things won't get done when they're around because they will either undo my work or get into trouble when I'm not watching them closely. But I've discovered that both of my older children absolutely *love* to be included in doing the housework.

Jude is thrilled whenever I ask him to help me unload the dishwasher. He also helps me load and unload the washer and dryer, and recently Jenesis decided she wanted to get in on the fun. I allow them both to push the buttons (under my watchful eye), and they think that's the greatest thing! Yes, it takes twice as long to do some things, but right now they are at an age where washing dishes with mommy is just as exciting as playing a game with me. Sure, down the road they probably won't always be as eager to help, but since I've allowed them to be part of my everyday tasks, they have reveled in being my "big helpers." Seeing their joyful faces beaming with the knowledge that they have been a help to me makes those few extra minutes worth it.

There's something in children that makes them feel valued and important when they are involved in the "big people" things of life. And when you think of it as an investment—both preparing them for more grown-up responsibilities as well as laying the foundation for their becoming capable, responsible adults—it really does become a joy to include them. This kind of approach will help tremendously when the new baby comes, because although the tasks may take longer, you know your children are eager to help.

Be Willing to Ask for Help

Near the end of my pregnancies, I have usually experienced excruciating nerve and back pain, which makes a lot of my normal cleaning tasks difficult. It's especially hard when I'm going through the nesting phase where I want everything to be sparkling before the baby arrives. A number of sweet friends offered help if I needed it, but during my first and second pregnancies I was too timid to take them up on it.

Finally, as my chores got really hard, my husband stepped in to ask if a couple of ladies would be willing to come in and do a bit of cleaning right before the birth. I was blown away by the reaction! These women went above and beyond to care for us and help ready our home for the arrival of the baby, and they made us feel loved in the process.

Don't hesitate to ask for help, *especially* if it's been offered. Our tendency as women can be to think that we're placing an extra burden on someone by asking for assistance. But put yourself in the other person's shoes for a moment. If you offer to help someone, don't you usually hope they'll take you up on it? It's a blessing both ways when we step out of our comfort zone and accept the help that's been offered.

Remember that although this is a difficult season—some say the most difficult—in a mother's life, it is also a season of great opportunity. Allow the Lord to stretch you and draw you closer to Him. Trust Him for wisdom and creativity, and He surely will delight to give it.

Our Appearance

As I mentioned earlier, I have received a number of surprising comments about my appearance while pregnant. Once I was walking (or waddling, rather) through the grocery store near the end of my second pregnancy and feeling very "great with child" when I paused in the floral department to enjoy the gorgeous blooms, as flowers are a weakness of mine. Then I felt a gentle touch on my arm and heard a woman's voice. I turned around to find a trim, well-dressed, middle-age woman whom I had never seen before.

I was slightly startled, but she quickly said, "I just wanted to tell you I was so surprised when you turned and I saw that you were expecting! You look so lovely! It's not normal to see expecting women with toddlers who are put together." I thanked her for her kind words before she moved on to another aisle.

This happened during my third trimester, when I was suffering from terrible back and nerve pain and really feeling those thirty-plus pounds of extra weight. I was quite tired and more than ready for that baby to come, so I was a bit shocked to receive such a compliment.

I had had the desire all through my teens and into marriage and motherhood to glorify God in my appearance—to reflect by how I carry myself outwardly the peace and order that Christ brings to my internal life. I don't mean that I dressed up to buy groceries or tried to look glamorous to get the oil changed in my car. Nevertheless, I did try to maintain the same standards of appearance whether pregnant or not.

Now, I'm not advocating for a specific style of dressing. Everyone has their own personal taste—some more classic, some more sporty, some leaning more toward business casual, others just casual. Your wardrobe ultimately matters little in the grand scheme of things. What *does* matter—and what will carry over into your style preferences—is that you aim for glorifying God in every area of your life, including your outward appearance.

Although the application is different from keeping a home, the foundational principle is the same. The way we present our bodies should be a reflection of the life of Jesus within us, just as keeping our homes should be.

In the women's ministry where I serve, we often receive inquiries about how important physical beauty should be in a Christian woman's life. The passage that is most often asked about in these conversations is 1 Peter 3:3–4, which reads, *"Do not let your adornment be merely outward—arranging the hair, wearing gold, or putting on fine apparel—rather let it be the hidden person of the heart, with the incorruptible beauty of a gentle and quiet spirit, which is very precious in the sight of God"* (NKJV).

Having been asked about this so many times, I decided to do some study on this passage of Scripture and what it really means. Was Peter saying that we should *not* braid our hair, put on gold jewelry, or wear nice clothing? Or does his admonition go deeper than that? After exploring the Word and considering this passage in light of the whole of Scripture, and seeking the counsel of my husband and godly older women, I've come to the conclusion that what this passage is really addressing is the condition of a person's heart.

There are other Scripture verses that certainly don't condemn the wearing of jewelry or nice clothing—Genesis 24:22–23; Exodus 28:2–6; Proverbs 31:21–22; and Song of Solomon 1:9–10, to name a few. But the governing principle that comes up over and over again is that God is *far* more concerned with the condition of our hearts—for example, see 1 Samuel 16:7; Matthew 23:25–27; and 2 Corinthians 5:12. Inevitably, what is inside us will overflow into every other aspect of our lives. How we care for our outward appearance is no exception.

I'm not talking about something that is necessarily legalistic. True, it's easy to fall into legalism when holding yourself (or others) to certain standards of modesty or only wearing styles that we consider feminine or ladylike. But this is something that is ultimately between a woman and God. I merely suggest that we attempt to carry ourselves in a way that reflects His beauty, His order, and His character.

I love this passage by Nancy DeMoss Wohlgemuth:

> *Nowhere does the Scripture condemn physical beauty or suggest that the outward appearance does not matter. What is condemned is taking pride in God-given beauty, giving excessive attention to physical beauty, or tending to physical matters while neglecting matters of the heart.*
>
> *One of Satan's strategies is to get us to move from one extreme to another. There is a growing aversion in our culture to neatness, orderliness, and attractiveness in*

dress and physical appearance. I sometimes find myself wanting to say to Christian women, "Do you know who you are? God made you a woman. Accept His gift. Don't be afraid to be feminine and to add physical and spiritual loveliness to the setting where He has placed you. You are a child of God. You are a part of the bride of Christ. You belong to the King—you are royalty. Dress and conduct yourself in a way that reflects your high and holy calling. God has called you out of this world's system—don't let the world press you into its mold. Don't think, dress, or act like the world; inwardly and outwardly, let others see the difference He makes in your life."[3]

I am not advocating that you go out and spend hundreds of dollars on an expensive maternity wardrobe, and I am not trying to pressure you into adopting a certain style of dress. What I am gently encouraging, though, is that during this season of pregnancy you carefully consider how you can dress in such a way that brings glory to God, displaying to this world that every aspect of who you are, both inside and out, is consecrated to the King of the universe.

Believe me, there have been many days when I made a run to the grocery store in sweatpants. But in those times, I still must remember who it is I represent and ask myself, *Am I dressing this way because it's practical for the situation, or am I just being lazy? Am I hasty and frazzled in my demeanor, or am I joyful and calm? Am I outward-focused, or am I thinking only of meeting my own needs? Am I impatient, or do I show grace to those around me?* Such questions can help us to gauge our hearts, because the answers have to do ultimately with that which sets us apart from the world. Clothing is just the icing on the cake.

For practical reasons, it can be hard to know how to go about building a maternity wardrobe after learning you're pregnant. Maternity clothes can be expensive, and not many moms-to-be have extra money lying around just waiting to be spent at A Pea in the Pod. But dressing in a fashion that honors God *can* be done well with some thoughtful planning. Here are a few practical suggestions that have helped me. I hope these will give you some ideas as you pray through how the Lord would want you to dress during this season.

Modesty

This is an important aspect to touch on since we're talking about Christians and clothing. While expecting my first, I was reading an informational book on pregnancy (written from a secular perspective) when I came to a section on dealing with enlarging breasts. After providing some helpful tips on how to be comfortable in your clothes, the section ended with a cringe-inducing line along the lines of "And since you now have more up there, take advantage of it and dare to wear those plunging necklines!"

If you will allow me to speak as one who has navigated these waters a few times, there seems to be a stronger temptation during pregnancy to wear clothes that are more revealing. Whether the motivation is insecurity about a husband's love, or the fact that everyone's focus is more on the baby than on the woman, or women simply want to feel better about themselves, I've noticed a growing trend in maternity photoshoots toward lower necklines, higher hemlines, and sometimes just undergarments.

Now, I know this is a touchy subject. And my goal is not to give you a heaping helping of guilt. What I do desire is to call all of us, as Christian women, to honor the Lord with our bodies, pregnant or not. Dressing in a way that is appropriately modest doesn't mean we are ashamed of our bodies. Rather, it's a reflection of our desire to honor the Lord and respect others. Scripture calls us to honor God with our bodies. Speaking in the context of sexual purity, Paul says in 1 Corinthians 6:19–20, "Or do you not know that your body is a temple of the Holy

Spirit within you, whom you have from God? You are not your own, for you were bought with a price. So glorify God in your body." In 1 Timothy 2:9, Paul speaks specifically of the need for modesty in a woman's clothing and accessories.

Christians' external appearance should give evidence of the life of Christ within us, and that is ultimately why dressing modestly is important. This has nothing to do with stodgy legalism and *everything* to do with the glory of God. That said, our approach to modesty should be "Will the clothing I wear be glorifying to Him?" rather than "How close can I get to the line without stepping over it?"

Even as our bellies expand and our clothes get tighter, and we have to forego wearing our favorite maternity top for the final few weeks because of it, we won't ever regret choosing God's glory over our style preferences.

God's Provision

I have heard (and experienced) some amazing stories of the Lord's provision in the simplest of things. Maternity clothing may seem like a funny thing to bring before the Lord in prayer, but remember, He is honored when we come to Him with even the smallest of petitions. He delights, as a Father, to provide for our every need. So start there, and you will be blessed and encouraged in your faith as you watch Him take care of every detail.

One of my favorite examples happened when I was looking for a maternity coat and went to my favorite secondhand shop, which often has a nice selection of maternity clothes. When I asked if they had any coats, I was told they didn't because they tend to sell quickly upon arrival. As I browsed the racks a bit before leaving, I overheard a lady come in who said she had some maternity clothes to sell. My ears perked up, and I peeked over at the counter to see what she had. Lo and behold, she pulled out a beautiful, camel-colored peacoat in wonderful condition.

I waited until she had left before running to the counter. "Did I just see a maternity coat come in?" I asked. Sure enough, it was exactly what I had been looking for—and in my size too! The shop girls couldn't stop talking about what a cool story this was, as I thanked the Lord for showing me His loving provision with something as simple as a coat.

Think Practically

More and more often, I hear and read about keeping a "capsule wardrobe." It basically means having a few pieces of clothing that can mix and match to create many different outfits. Without realizing it, that is what I did when I began choosing maternity clothing. I've now been through four pregnancies, and I still wear pretty much everything I got the first time around. What I have found is that the items I've worn least are the things that go with only one other item of clothing.

A few more tips along these lines: Choose colors that you know you'll want to wear often. Choose styles that you feel comfortable in. And be sure you have a *few* things to wear for special occasions. You never know when you'll be invited to a wedding that takes place when you're seven months pregnant. Even so, these dressy pieces can be practical and versatile—in other words, choose something you can wear in both summer and winter.

Buy Secondhand and Borrow from Friends

Most of my favorite maternity pieces have come from second-hand stores. Pre-owned maternity clothes are usually in great condition since they've been worn for only a few months, and they are far less expensive than buying new. My two favorite places to shop for secondhand clothing are Clothes Mentor (a chain with stores across the U.S.) and an online thrift store called ThredUP.

Several friends have let me borrow their maternity clothes when they're not using them. This is a really great way to save money and have some fun, new things to wear for the next several months.

Get Creative with Your Non-Maternity Clothes

In my second pregnancy I discovered that one of my favorite things to do was wear a cardigan or button-down shirt open, with a solid maternity T-shirt underneath and a thin belt above my bump. It felt put-together but was very comfortable at the same time. Also, non-maternity camisoles and high-necked tank tops are much less expensive than the maternity versions. And when you wear them to add more coverage to shirts that may be lacking, it doesn't really matter how tight they are since they'll be worn underneath.

While you're being creative with your wardrobe, don't forget to have fun with accessories. Scarves, fun earrings, hats, necklaces—whatever you enjoy. These little touches can brighten a plain outfit and make it feel special.

Remember Who You Are

Remember in all these things—your home, your clothing, and other visible aspects of your life—that the goal is to glorify Jesus. It's not to get your home on the cover of *Martha Stewart Living* or to be featured in a Motherhood Maternity ad. You will have days when the house is less than perfect and you go to the mailbox while wearing yesterday's mascara and pajama bottoms. But if you will continually submit the practical areas of your life to the Lord, He will give you wisdom, creativity, and joy and help with every detail of caring for your body and the home He has given you.

Testimony from a Godly Mama

LAUREN
Mother of Two

Think of the work of being a mom as a sacred responsibility from the Lord. Why? Because just like anything else He has given you—life, talents, home, marriage, and more—the responsibility of mothering is certainly intended to bless you, but it's mostly to glorify Him.

The everyday experience of raising children is such that one moment finds you soaring high on the joy of hearing your baby's first laugh, yet that same hour you find yourself fighting tears when you realize that your favorite pre-pregnancy jeans still don't fit your soft, postpartum body. Motherhood brings with it moments of incredible poignancy and emotional highs and lows, but it is also very ... normal.

Wake kids and snuggle on the couch. Make breakfast. Remind one child to be thankful for her "yucky" oatmeal and the other child to use his spoon, not his hands, to eat. Read together from the Bible and experience a heart-swelling moment when one child asks you a surprisingly profound spiritual question. Send the kids off to play while you eyeball the pile of dishes waiting in the sink.

Colossians 3:23–24 tells us:
> *Whatever you do, work heartily, as*
> *for the Lord and not for men, knowing*
> *that from the Lord you will receive*
> *the inheritance as your reward.*
> *You are serving the Lord Christ.*

"Whatever you do" includes every moment of being a mom. It means embracing the discomforts of pregnancy in order to birth new life, and choosing to rejoice instead of complain when you wake (again) to a fussing baby at 2 a.m. It also means mopping up sticky spills, mediating sibling squabbles, and making sure everyone in the family has clean clothes.

Before we are wives and mothers, we are simply women before the Lord—women created for the purpose of bringing praise and glory to Him in every area of our lives. Motherhood is a gift from God, given that He may use it to make us more like Him while revealing His character and nature in the everyday tasks of nurturing, tending, and teaching.

When our attention wanders and we lose focus on the glory of God, it's easy to become mired in the seeming mundanity of caring for home and family and wonder, *What's the point of all this endless work?* On the flip side, when everything's going smoothly and we're feeling like Supermom, we can easily fall prey to the pride of mothering with excellence, as though the point of it all is merely to satisfy our own goals and desires. As we seek to be faithful stewards of our homes and children, the knowledge that we are serving our worthy Lord must be what propels us forward, not just the sheer necessity of the work or our desire for personal fulfillment.

So on those days when you manage to savor a glorious hour of quiet time with the Lord before the kids get up, your hair is on point, and the dishes get washed after every meal … aim your heart toward Jesus and His glory. And on the days when you are frantically whipping your hair into a messy bun, wearing yesterday's jeans, and hurrying off to the pediatrician with a feverish baby ... aim your heart toward Jesus and His glory. You will find Him more than faithful to walk with you along every step of your mothering journey.

8

PREGNANCY AND SERVICE

And having a reputation for good works: if she has
brought up children, has shown hospitality, has
washed the feet of the saints, has cared for the afflicted,
and has devoted herself to every good work.
1 Timothy 5:10

March 14, 2015. I had been anticipating this date for nine long months. Now I found myself waiting at the hospital where I would give birth to our third child—only not on this day. I was there for a different reason. A friend of ours, who lives in our home, woke up that morning needing to visit the ER. It all felt very surreal. I had gotten very little sleep the last two long weeks because I was having contractions every ten minutes around the clock. At this moment, I wanted more than anything to be admitted to this hospital and give birth to my daughter, but God had a different plan for me. And it struck me that today—my due date—was really a culmination of something the Lord had started forming in my life during my second pregnancy: selfless service.

Two months before our second child was born, my mother-in-law returned from the mission field to have testing done for some health issues she was having. We have an amazing healthcare facility nearby, and it made so much sense for her to stay with us, which would also give our son Jude time to spend with Grandma. Her doctors discovered she had an aggressive form of cancer, and they immediately started her on chemotherapy. With the devastating news, my father-in-law and my husband's two younger siblings also flew back to be with her through this difficult time. Suddenly, we had a very full house, and we all lived in close quarters for the next three months. There was a significant adjustment period as we figured out how two families—who are all part of the same family—could function in a complementary way for an extended period of time while walking through incredibly difficult circumstances.

I must admit, I gave in to selfishness far too many times during those three months—mostly because my own expectations weren't being met—and I often struggled with the smallest of details. Earlier in that second pregnancy, I had begun praying that the Lord would teach me what it meant to be selfless and servant-hearted and ready at any moment to serve those whom God brought into our lives. Now here He was, walking me through a refining process (with many tears of repentance) and challenging me: Was I willing to unconditionally serve others, laying down my own expectations and "needs" when I was so close to my due date?

In that season, the Lord taught me that my pregnancy and the smooth functioning of my little family were not what was most important. Here was my mother-in-law, walking through one of the most challenging seasons of her life, and I was per-turbed that someone had put my saucepan away in the wrong cupboard. That put things into perspective quickly. I knew that I may never have another opportunity to spend time with my in-laws or show them love and hospitality in such a unique way, and I wanted to do it well.

Things really turned around in my heart from that point forward. To be sure, I didn't handle everything perfectly. This was a growing process, but they extended so much grace to me. Truly, you couldn't ask for better people to share your home with for that amount of time, and I have thanked God for them many times. I pray I will never forget the things I learned in that season.

Hospitality: Service in Action

One of the important ways Christians are called to serve others is through hospitality. Webster's 1828 dictionary defines *hospitality* as:

> *The act or practice of receiving and entertaining strangers or guests without reward, or with kind and generous liberality.*

This sounds about right. The apostle Peter commands us, "Show hospitality to one another without grumbling. As each has received a gift, use it to serve one another, as good stewards of God's varied grace" (1 Peter 4:9–10). Paul says simply, "Contribute to the needs of the saints and seek to show hospitality" (Romans 12:13).

Biblical hospitality means more than throwing an occasional holiday party or baby shower or hosting a visiting missionary. Hospitality is a way of life, an attitude that puts others above ourselves and is ready at all times to show love to those whom God brings across our paths, however inconvenient the timing. As I mentioned in the previous chapter, it's not about keeping a pristine home, and it's not about cooking a gourmet meal whenever there's company. Goldfish crackers and water may be the only things in the house you can offer a visitor, but if they are offered in genuine care for your guest, it can be far more meaningful than the most elaborate meal.

I love how Jen Wilkin, author of *Women of the Word*, describes the difference between entertaining and hospitality:

Entertaining involves setting the perfect tablescape after an exhaustive search on Pinterest. It chooses a menu that will impress, and then frets its way through each stage of preparation. It requires every throw pillow to be in place, every cobweb to be eradicated, every child to be neat and orderly. It plans extra time to don the perfect outfit before the first guest touches the doorbell on the seasonally decorated doorstep. And should any element of the plan fall short, entertaining perceives the entire evening to have been tainted. Entertaining focuses attention on self.

Hospitality involves setting a table that makes everyone feel comfortable. It chooses a menu that allows face time with guests instead of being chained to the stovetop. It picks up the house to make things pleasant, but doesn't feel the need to conceal evidences of everyday life. It sometimes sits down to dinner with flour in its hair. It allows the gathering to be shaped by the quality of the conversation rather than the cuisine. Hospitality shows interest in the thoughts, feelings, pursuits, and preferences of its guests. It is good at asking questions and listening intently to answers. Hospitality focuses attention on others.[1]

I love Jen's point. Hospitality means being outward-focused, not trying to draw attention to our cooking or hosting skills. It's not wrong to have these skills or work to cultivate them, but they are to be a means of blessing others and not just the point of having someone over for dinner.

Of course, true hospitality isn't always easy. Actually, it's often difficult and involves some degree of sacrifice. It sometimes means saying yes last minute to having someone stay the night (or two or three or *lots* of nights). It will sometimes mean inviting into your personal space people who are not sensitive to your time or how you run your home. Other times it might mean spending more on groceries than you anticipated, requiring you to trim other areas of your budget that month.

Whatever the case, we must always be ready and willing to obediently show hospitality as God calls us. Hebrews 13:2 reminds us, "Do not neglect to show hospitality to strangers, for thereby some have entertained angels unawares." Remember, the momentary sacrifices you make will reap eternal reward. We may never see that reward in *this* life, but we can be sure that God is pleased and honored when we choose an eternal focus over a temporal one.

Living in this way can be especially significant during a season of pregnancy. We are used to hearing that pregnancy is a time to look inward and focus on our bodies and ourselves, so showing hospitality and serving able-bodied individuals may go against what seems normal or even right. But women who maintain an outward focus—extending hospitality even when they're more physically taxed—stand out in displaying the supernatural love and grace of Jesus whatever their circumstances. During pregnancy, we may be more limited in the range of our service, but if we allow the Lord to use us to bless others, it will most certainly have an impact on those who see.

Leaving a Legacy of Service

I have been so blessed to inherit a multigenerational vision for servant-hearted hospitality. My mom and dad both come from families that made it a high priority. When my mom's family first joined their home church more than thirty years ago, my dad's family was the first to have them over for dinner. Both families shared their home (and still do) with missionaries and others in need for weeks or months at a time. They were always prepared to make food stretch as far as need be to accommodate anyone who might sit at their table at any given meal. And even though both sets of parents are now in their eighties, they are still always looking for ways to serve the people around them. Our parents are beloved by all who know them, and that is no exaggeration.

In my very early years, we had several foreign exchange students live in our home, and we often had people we barely knew over for meals. Our move to Mongolia when I was seven years old didn't change this. My parents had earned a reputation for being the ones everyone called upon for help, the ones to take in kids when their missionary parents had a medical emergency and had to leave the country, and the ones who spent money on imported foods for a special meal just to let their guests know they were loved. Our friends sometimes assumed we were wealthy because of things like that, but the truth is, we had no more than most missionaries we've known. My parents simply chose to invest in those things that others might find frivolous to be a means of blessing and refreshment to those who were giving so much to bless others.

It was because of my parent's hospitality that we got to know my husband and his family so well. They had lived in Mongolia for just under two years when Judah's brother was in a near-fatal horseback accident and had to be evacuated by air to receive proper medical care. We didn't know them well at the time, but my parents didn't hesitate to offer their home for Judah and his two youngest siblings to stay as long as needed. So today we have a little family joke that God had to use a horse to bring us together. But seriously, from that point on, our families became very dear friends. You never know how one act of service might change the course of someone's life.

My mom gave birth to two children during the time we lived in Mongolia. I can't remember a single instance during either pregnancy (including one that was high-risk) when she stopped opening our home to others. This was despite learning to shop in a language that was not her own and living in a small apartment with multiple kids and a very tiny kitchen. (The top of our washing machine was the kitchen "counter" in our first apartment.) Once a week for nearly two years, a Mongolian family who didn't have running water came over to take showers in our home. Guests slept on our living room floor when they came from out of town. I could go on, but this should give you a pretty good idea of the selfless way my mother served and gave of herself, even in circumstances that most of us would consider less than ideal. But my mother's focus was on eternity, not her immediate surroundings. Yes, there were difficult moments when I could tell her life wasn't all rainbows and butterflies. Her chosen life required sacrifice. But because her eyes were fixed on Jesus, she was able to minister in the capacity the Lord had planned for her, and many, many lives were touched as a result.

Because of our families' example of practicing intentional, sacrificial, Christ-exalting hospitality, my husband and I are committed to carrying on this legacy in our home. When I was pregnant for the second time, we felt the need to begin praying a very specific prayer: for the Lord to provide a place to expand our family and our hospitality. Very shortly after we began praying, God provided an absolutely beautiful home for us to rent for almost two years, and during that time, we had more than fifty people stay for a night or more (not including those who visited just for a meal). We knew that this was one of the biggest reasons God had provided this home for us.

It wasn't always easy, having two young children and some-times back-to-back company arriving (when I was already running behind on any number of tasks). In fact, there were many times I lay in my bed at night wondering how in the world I was going to do yet another day. But that is where the vision for hospitality comes in. I had to keep in mind the fact that God calls us to show service to others in this way, and He gives me everything I need to accomplish it.

Now we want to pass this vision on to our children. We can see how our parents' obedience in showing hospitality has greatly affected our view of it, and we want the same for our kids. Already, we can see the effects in their lives. All of our children are very different in nature, but when visitors enter our home, all the children enthusiastically welcome them. We have had so many guests in our home that it doesn't faze them when someone they've never seen walks through our door. And when we are out and about, they greet everyone they see. The surprised delight on the faces of the people we pass in the store is beautiful to behold. My children are learning a lifestyle of hospitality that we hope and pray will open many doors for them to one day share the gospel with others.

You may be thinking, *I didn't have that kind of legacy passed down to me. I've never seen practical examples of this kind of hospitality, so is this even possible for me?* The answer is yes. Ultimately, it doesn't matter whether or not you grew up in such a home. Even if you are a first-generation Christian, you have an opportunity to open up your heart and home because God's enabling grace surpasses experience. His Spirit can teach you what hospitality looks like for you, and He will help you to start a legacy to pass along to your own children. And if you're expecting a child while reading this book, now is the perfect time to start!

Practical Hospitality: What Does It Look Like for Me?

I believe the Lord calls every Christian to varying levels of hospitality, and He gives to each of us particular giftings to be used for service. Some of us are called to open our homes to many people, while others will be called to different forms of hospitality and service. But I do want to challenge your heart in this matter. Are you willing to give up some comfort and convenience and adherence to a strict schedule in order to welcome others into your family's home and lives? Are you willing to allow the Lord to use you in this way as an instrument of grace in the lives of others?

Each of us is responsible before the Lord to be obedient to the leadings He places on our hearts. When you begin to look around at the many needs in just your community, it's easy to become overwhelmed by the sheer number of ways you could show hospitality to others. Remember that it is not more "spiritual" to burn yourself out by saying yes to every single opportunity that comes your way. According to Ephesians 2:10, you were created in Christ Jesus to do *specific* good works that God has prepared especially for you that you should walk in them.

Long ago He planned particular ways for you to minister to the people in your community and within your sphere of influence. These may be as simple as taking a meal to a family whose mom has just given birth. Or it may mean taking in a family who is without a home for a period of time. Pray and trust that the Lord will give you clear direction as needs arise and that His Spirit will give you the grace, the desire, and the power to do what pleases Him.

In the meantime, here are some practical considerations as you seek what God has planned for you in this season.

Know Your Calling

It's not optional for Christians to show hospitality; it's a command to all of us. But to what extent we are called is something that is unique to each individual. Bring this before the Lord, and then walk in obedience as He brings opportunities into your path. And whatever He asks of you, step forward in obedience without hesitation, no matter how new or daunting the task may appear. You will find that you are given all the grace you need, "for it is God who works in you, both to will and to work for his good pleasure" (Philippians 2:13).

Know Your Limits

One thing we discovered about making our home so open to others is that we were constantly being presented with opportunities to reach out. And at times, we didn't stop to think whether or not it was the prudent thing to do. We simply said, "Sure, those days are open, so why not?" But the things that God was *not* actually asking of us soon became apparent, as the unnecessary strain these put on our family was made abundantly clear.

So be wise and discerning as "opportunities" arise to determine whether they are for you or someone else to take up. This is not to say there won't be times when the Holy Spirit calls you to sacrifice your comfort or schedule to show love to someone in need. But you need to prayerfully evaluate and seek the Lord's wisdom for each situation.

Know Your Season

There will be seasons in your life when you are called to to be more or less active in ministry. For instance, if you are a pregnant woman on bed rest, chances are the Lord is not calling you to volunteer for every available service opportunity. Or, as you are preparing to welcome a little one, the Spirt may be prompting you to intentionally invest more time in your marriage and children, so that your home is well prepared to bring another life into the mix.

Remember, it's what God is asking of you that's important, not the expectations of others. If you're like me, you may feel self-imposed pressure to take on more than you should out of fear of what other people might think if you say no. Or you might find yourself saying yes too often out of a desire for applause and recognition. Both are selfishly motivated and will never reap good fruit.

Just before we welcomed our third child, we purchased a home that is quite a bit smaller than the one we had been renting previously. This forced us to reevaluate what hospitality would look like practically for us in the future. We could no longer have as many people stay in our home, because we had lost the extra guest room. During this transition, we felt the Lord asking us to pull back the reins on our outside ministry for the sake of investing more time and attention in our children, especially as it pertained to growing them spiritually. We knew the Lord wanted our family to be strong and ready to minister effectively in the coming years, and for each of our children to thrive and participate in the approaching seasons of ministry.

Seasons of pulling back, refocusing, and preparing are as vital to your effectiveness in service and ministry as your willingness and desire to pour yourself out on behalf of others. So know your season and walk in it with confidence, even if it means resting in the Lord and regrouping for a time.

Know Your Environment

Preparing a hospitable atmosphere in your home starts with seeking the Lord and asking Him to cultivate His love, peace, joy, and selflessness in the very core of your being, for the attitude of your heart will play a huge part in how guests experience your hospitality.

My grandparents' home is called Peace Cottage, and it has lived up to that name lo these many years. So many times people have said to me, "I love being in your grandparents' home! There's just something different about it. I can't really explain it." This was true of my parents' home, and Judah and I pray that it is true of our home as well. What is the secret? My family has made a commitment to keep Christ at the center of our lives and homes.

Jesus is our reason for being, the One who made us and for whom we were made. Everything we do should give God glory and proclaim the praises of the risen King who called us out of darkness into His wonderful light (1 Peter 2:9). As His ambassadors to the world, we are meant to reflect the Son's light into the lives of everyone around us, and hospitality is an impactful way of doing that.

Keep in mind, however, that you can own the most beautiful home with the loveliest furnishings and serve the most incredible food, but if the Spirit of the Lord isn't present there, then your home will be missing what your guests need most. Yes, you can still bless them with a clean, tastefully decorated home and an excellent meal, but if your motivation for providing these things is to give a flawless performance or to win the praises of your guests instead of glorifying Christ, then it is ultimately an empty gesture.

Know Your Vision

It is important to Judah and me that our children see and experience the incredible joy that comes from extending hospitality to others. We don't want our children to look back on these years and think, *Dad and Mom were always ministering to others and never had time for us kids.* Both Judah and I had parents with extensive hospitality ministries, but rather than feeling neglected as children, we felt like active participants in our parents' service to others. I can't begin to count how many times we would be preparing to have a new family over for dinner and my dad would gather us kids together and say, "We are going to be a blessing to this family." That was a commission we didn't take lightly.

When you share with your children a vision for the beauty that comes from ministering to others, they won't resent it but will instead embrace it as their calling too. Invite your children into your plans. Let them help with preparing meals, making beds, or picking flowers for the table. Talk with them about the excitement of having people in your home and what a privilege and a joy it is to extend Christ's love to others. Share Bible verses with them about hospitality, even if your children are young.

Trust the Holy Spirit to impress the truth on their hearts and minds as you faithfully impart it to them.

Even if you are expecting your first child, you can still share a vision for hospitality by inviting others to participate in your pregnancy. It's very tempting to isolate ourselves during this emotionally fragile time, but I have heard from others how thankful they were that I allowed them to share in both the beauties and difficulties of my pregnancy. Inviting family, friends, and neighbors into the joy of this time, even if it feels a little uncomfortable at first, will expand your own joy while giving others an opportunity to love and serve you.

When You're Feeling Less than Hospitable

The ministry of hospitality is a beautiful one. You never know how a simple act of service might impact someone's life for eternity. But what about those times when you're feeling like the one in need of service?

Remember that it is often when we feel at our weakest that the Lord's power may be perfected in our lives (2 Corinthians 12:9–10). When you make the choice to serve out of the little you feel you have to offer, God will take your service to Him and expand it far beyond your natural capacity.

I will give Elisabeth Elliot the final word on this subject:

> Do you often feel like parched ground, unable to produce anything worthwhile? I do. When I am in need of refreshment, it isn't easy to think of the needs of others. But I have found that if, instead of praying for my own comfort and satisfaction, I ask the Lord to enable me to give to others, an amazing thing often happens—I find my own needs wonderfully met. Refreshment comes in ways I would never have thought of, both for others, and then, incidentally, for myself.[2]

Testimony from a Servant-Hearted Mama

TRINA
Mother of Four

Bending down over my growing pregnant belly to pick up half-full cups of tobacco spit to keep our newly mobile toddler from accidentally ingesting the nasty brown slime—this did not exactly fit into my dreamy vision of what warmhearted hospitality looked like. But taking in my wayward brother and his best friend in hopes of seeing their lives impacted by Jesus Christ did.

Through the years, my husband and I have seen the many faces of hospitality: Housing a homeless man in a makeshift apartment on our southern Ohio farm. Hosting a U.S. ambassador, an army general, and a British actor in our tent on the Mongolian mission field. Turning our twenty-four-square-foot cabin into a temporary hotel for a dozen disabled Mongol children so that their parents could afford to bring them to their nation's most cherished national park.

High on the apostle Paul's list of qualifications for a bishop of the church is to be given to hospitality (1 Timothy 3:1–7). To "give" yourself to biblical hospitality does not mean merely having an occasional guest over for dinner. Rather, I like to think of hospitality as a continual posture of outstretched arms extending invitations and being ready to lovingly receive people, whether for an evening meal, a small Bible study, a game night, a weekend stay, or long-term living when needed.

Speaking of the kind of hospitality admonished in Romans 12:13, John Piper says that the phrasing of this verse literally means to "pursue hospitality" and implies "continuous action." It's just not just a once-a-year thing at Thanksgiving or Christmas but is a "constant attitude and practice."[3] Such ongoing seasons of ministering to our neighbors or entertaining strangers will certainly require times of quiet rest to refuel as a family. But the biblical mandate to be lovers of hospitality is an indisputable duty and should be a consistent characteristic of every Spirit-filled follower of Christ.

The country of Mongolia, where we have lived and ministered for the last fifteen years, is known for the hospitable nature of her nomadic herdsmen. The word **privacy** does not even exist in the Mongolian language, and the concept of personal property is hardly evident in their community-oriented countryside culture. It is as natural as breathing for modest families living in a yurt—a portable, felt-covered tent—to gladly make room on their wood pallet floors to lay out extra mats for family, friends, and passing strangers.

In our early days in the field, we had the difficult daily task of hauling water from the village's pristine mountain lake for drinking and to use in bathing, cooking, and washing dishes and clothes. One such morning, forever etched in my mind, was when three young Jewish men passing through town knocked on our door. They asked if this was a guest house and where they might do some laundry. I was tempted to send them down the road, saying, "No, I am sorry, this is a private home." But the still small voice of the

Spirit whispered to my heart, "Take them in, make them a meal, and clean their laundry." Over the course of the afternoon, these simple gestures opened the door for us to introduce these men to the glorious gospel of their Messiah, and we gave each one of them a copy of the New Testament in their native Hebrew tongue.

We cherish that sweet memory among so many others of the wonderful people the Lord has brought to our home in the northern Mongolian tundra. And though I cannot say that I have always shown hospitality "without grudging" as 1 Peter 4:9 tells us to do, I can honestly proclaim that we have never regretted allowing God to increase our capacity to love others in this way. What a blessing to have experienced the ongoing, overflowing joy that comes through sacrificial service!

9

Pregnancy and Community

*God has so composed the body ... that there may be no
division in the body, but that the members may have the
same care for one another. If one member suffers, all suffer
together; if one member is honored, all rejoice together.*
1 Corinthians 12:24–26

One evening, midway through my fourth pregnancy, I received a phone call from a woman in our church. After just a minute or two of exchanging pleasantries, she told me the reason for her call. "Judah told me Sunday that you've been having a harder time physically with this pregnancy. I was wondering if you would let me set up a meal schedule for you for a few weeks to help lighten the load?" I was completely surprised, as the thought of something like that hadn't even entered my mind. Even so, I knew it was a direct answer to prayer.

This had been an intense season in our lives, particularly on the ministry side of things. As much as I loved hosting people in our home, I could tell my energy was steadily diminishing, as even the simplest tasks of keeping a home were becoming difficult to manage. The day before the phone call, I was sitting in my favorite corner of our bedroom, looking out the window as I rocked in our glider. I prayed and asked the Lord for grace and strength to do what He had called me to do, because I had no idea how I was going to keep up at the pace our lives were moving. But God chose to the address the issue in a much more practical way than I had expected. What I didn't know was that my health was about to go downhill significantly in the days to come, and those meals would be an incredible and welcome provision.

In my pride, I was very tempted to graciously decline the offer, thinking about the many other church families whose babies had been and would be arriving in the days to come. Simply put, I didn't want to feel like I was being a burden to others. But as this precious woman reminded me in a text a few days later, "That's what the body of Christ is for!" I knew then I needed to humbly accept this as a gift from my loving heavenly Father.

We Need Each Other

American culture places a high value on independence and self-reliance. We pride ourselves on being able to do things on our own, and we see it as weakness when we must accept help from our neighbors. Even when we desperately need assistance, we would often rather suffer under the weight of the burden than humble ourselves and ask for help. This mindset has even found its way into the church; it's often subconscious but there nonetheless.

This is not how God intended for us to live. He didn't create people to be independent but, rather, *interdependent*. From the beginning, He designed us to live in community, helping and encouraging one another as a way of demonstrating the love of God to our neighbors and to a watching world. After all, people are made in the image of the One who has lived eternally in perfect, harmonious relationship as three persons in one—Father, Son, and Holy Spirit.

Even in the Land of Rugged Individualism, the church is meant to model the spirit of interdependence and cooperation. Jesus said, "By this all people will know that you are my disciples, if you have love for one another" (John 13:35). There is no way we can hope to display this kind of love for one another—the kind of self-sacrificial love that will make unbelievers stop and stare in awe—if we are not living in intentional, life-giving community with those whom God has placed around us in our local church body. We must be ready and willing not only to enter into other people's lives, but to allow them into ours as well. This takes vulnerability and humility and isn't without risk. But it is this kind of love that will witness to the world about the God we serve.

I don't know about you, but I am one of those people who is much more comfortable being on the giving end of a need than on the receiving end. I have always taken to heart Jesus' teaching that "it is more blessed to give than to receive" (Acts 20:35). However, the Lord has used pregnancy to show me that in order for there to be a giver, there must also be a receiver; for someone to meet a need, there must be someone with a need to be met. And I cannot deny that when pregnant, I am more likely to be the one in the position of need. It's a humbling place to be, yet God allows us to be in this position of need in order to strengthen the body of Christ, and we must be willing to accept the service of others in the name of Jesus.

Paul writes in Galatians 6:2, "Bear one another's burdens, and so fulfill the law of Christ." When we alongside our brothers and sisters in Christ, encouraging and helping one another, we are actually fulfilling the law of Christ. So it goes without saying that if this isn't happening, then we are falling short in obeying Him. This can happen in one of two ways: Either we see a need that we should be filling but choose not to, or we refuse to allow others to help us. Either way, the driving motivation behind our actions is not love, but selfishness, pride, or fear.

Godly community during pregnancy or any other season of life is an incredible gift from the Lord. Yet sadly, we have all seen or heard stories of the body of Christ being more hurtful than helpful, more life-taking than life-giving. Each of us needs to ask the Lord to show us in what ways we need to repent of our own failings, and what steps we need to take to in order to walk in obedience to foster a loving, caring community with our brothers and sisters in Christ.

Remember, the little one you're expecting will be joining not only a biological family, but also a larger, spiritual family. It is our responsibility as parents to demonstrate for our children that this relationship requires us both to serve our spiritual brothers *and* to humbly and gratefully allow them to contribute to our needs and help bear our burdens when that is the position we are in.

There have been many ways in which members of God's family have come alongside me to help when I was pregnant. Sometimes the help was of a practical nature, such as the time when a group of single ladies from our church offered to come and do a thorough house cleaning for us. Other times help has been of a spiritual and emotional nature. During my third pregnancy, I was going through a really tough season emotionally, so one of my dear friends made time to check in on me and pray with me. She would also send me scriptures to meditate on and sermons to listen to. One mother sent her older daughter over for a couple of hours once a week to watch the kids so I could get a little bit of extra rest or work done.

In each of these situations, and others, I could have easily declined and was tempted to do so. But it would have been only pride that kept me from accepting the practical outpouring of Christ's love that compelled these precious people to give of their time, energy, and resources to care for me and my family. And every time, it has proven to be exactly what I needed.

Sadly, many moms don't have this kind of community surrounding and supporting them, for various reasons. Sometimes it's because their family is not involved in a local church community, but other times the church they attend isn't fully doing their job of being the body. In both of these situations, something needs to change.

If your family is not engaging regularly in fellowship with a local church body, I greatly encourage you to begin doing so right away—first, out of obedience to Christ (Hebrews 10:24–25), and second, because God has given us the body of Christ not only for His glory but also for our good (Ecclesiastes 4:9–1; 1 Corinthians 12:24–26). We are not meant to live the Christian life in isolation. When we do, we cut ourselves off from a significant source of grace, love, and encouragement.

Do Unto Others

If you are in a situation where the church body you are a part of isn't modeling this kind of love and the servant heart of Jesus, my first encouragement would be to pray for your church—pray that the Lord would raise up among the people a heart of love toward one another. Second, I would encourage you to remember Jesus' words: "Whatever you wish that others would do to you, do also to them" (Matthew 7:12). Model the kind of love and care you yearn to have others offer to you in times of need. If you're in the midst of a difficult season, your efforts may need to be on a simple level, but look for opportunities to model love in action in whatever ways you are able.

I mentioned earlier that my fourth pregnancy was quite difficult, and I had some stretches where I wasn't able to do much of anything and relied quite a bit on others. However, there was one day I was at the grocery store shortly after a baby had been born to another family in our church, and I remembered what a blessing it had been to me when people had brought over little, "special" things to munch on between meals. So I grabbed a few items before checking out and dropped them off with this newly blessed family on my way home. Even though I wasn't able to make a full meal, I was able to provide them an unexpected treat. It doesn't have to be big to communicate love.

Humble Yourself

It can be incredibly humbling to ask someone to come clean your bathrooms or help you cook a meal or watch your kids while you take a nap. But it's this kind of vulnerability and willingness to allow others to help that builds deep love and trust amongst God's people. This is a wonderful thing to be able to foster.

There are so many "one another" passages in the New Testament, and these can only be lived out if we are doing life with other people. Don't feel guilty about needing help. God will give you the grace to receive it, just as He will give you opportunities to show love and serve others in return when the time comes. But trust that He is using your time of weakness to bring greater strength and unity to His body, and in so doing, He is being glorified.

EMILY
Mother of One

Strange fact: I broke my pinky toe about three months ago. I learned then that when one part of the body is injured or immobilized, the whole body is affected. Indeed, my whole body seemed to be in pain after breaking my little toe, probably because I was walking funny for a while afterward.

I have also experienced the joy and heartache that comes with sharing life with a local church community. What a precious witness of our faith it is when we act as one body, loving and caring for our own while enabling and encouraging one another to thrive!

We have been blessed with two pregnancies—one that bore the fruit of a healthy child, and one that ended in the pain-filled sorrow of losing a life too soon. Our first pregnancy brought us our daughter, Corrie Hope. She announced her presence at the exact same time we had said yes to fostering a one-month-old baby boy. We had nine months to prep for Corrie. She was planned for; he was not. We had less than three weeks from the time we heard of his existence to when we held him in our arms. Because of the short notice, we had absolutely NO baby things. Not one single thing.

We sent an e-mail to our church family explaining the situation, and within one week we had four full crates of baby clothes and diapers that would last for the eight months that he'd be staying with us.

Now *that* is testimony of provision! The fatherless was clothed because we were vulnerable enough to say we needed help.

Nine months after my daughter was born, we found out we were expecting again. Excited, we shared the news with our closest circle of friends very early on. We knew this was unconventional, but we were too joyful not to share. Then a few days later, I found I was bleeding.

In complete shock, we hesitantly set up an appointment the next day and texted our circle of close friends, who we knew would be praying with us. The bleeding got worse, and the doctor confirmed the miscarriage. We were numb.

We took a long while to fully grasp what it meant and how God could allow this. But through those first few months of sorrow, we received a constant flow of life, truth, and love through our brothers and sisters in Christ. At one point, every counter in our little home was covered with flowers and notes of comfort and truth. The baby had lived only five weeks in my womb, and yet even this smallest life was celebrated.

We felt strongly the need to share our loss with the rest of the church and acknowledge the life that God gave. Our oneness with these dear people only grew as we welcomed them into the deepest sorrow we had ever known.

There is an extremely vulnerable aspect to pregnancy: the realization as a mother that you are not in control. You can either recognize that vulnerability and allow it to bond you to your community of family and friends, or you can do the exact opposite and hide yourself away, refraining from functioning at all within the community. I strongly encourage you to let the gift of your pregnancy bring life to many. You have been blessed to be a blessing (2 Corinthians 9:11). Your gift, whatever the outcome, is meant to be given. May Christ be ever more celebrated in your life through each story He gives you to draw you closer to Him and His people!

10

PREGNANCY AND PREPARING FOR LABOR

*But he said to me, "My grace is sufficient for you,
for my power is made perfect in weakness." There-
fore I will boast all the more gladly of my weaknesses,
so that the power of Christ may rest upon me.*
2 Corinthians 12:9

My mom was pregnant with her fourth child at the time. We had recently moved, and she'd befriended one of our new neighbors from across the street. The neighbor and her husband were not believers, and she was very closed to talking about anything having to do with Christianity. She had two adopted children, but she was not able to have children of her own, which pained her deeply. At some point, she told my mother it had been a dream of hers to witness a birth. My mom began feeling the Lord's prompting to ask this woman to be present at the upcoming birth of my brother. Mom was at first hesitant to do so, as she is a very private person and had only ever allowed my dad and her mother with her in the delivery room. But she continued to feel pressed by the Lord to invite this woman in, and so she did.

All my mother's other labors had gone smoothly with no complications. But this one was different. Everything went well up until a few moments after my brother had been delivered. There was an issue with the placenta, and Mom began hemorrhaging badly. Things became very intense as the blood transfusion team was readied and the surgeon prepared for the possibility of an emergency hysterectomy. All the while, with our neighbor witnessing, my parents clung to the Lord and His peace. Thankfully, the bleeding subsided before more drastic measures were needed, and my mother was able to avoid a hysterectomy. (She would give birth to four more children in the years to come.)

Due to blood loss, Mom was put on bed rest for a couple of weeks while she regained her strength. Within a few days of being discharged from the hospital, she received a call from our neighbor, who said, "I know you're not really supposed to see anyone right now, but I have to talk with you." That day, our neighbor told her she had never seen anything like the way my parents walked calmly and peacefully through that life-or-death situation. She told my mom, "I need what you have," and she gave her life to the Lord that day.

Tears fill my eyes as I recall this story. Because of how my mom endured her most difficult labor and delivery, this woman who had been so opposed to the gospel surrendered her life to Jesus. This had a profound impact on me and has given me a vision for how the Lord desires to use the marvel of childbirth for His glory.

When I wrote this chapter, I was eight weeks from the due date of my third child and have since had my fourth. With every pregnancy, I am reminded afresh of the truths the Lord has taught me during the preparation for each of my deliveries. Still, after going through it three times, it was amazing how those butterflies came back as I planned for the fourth. Yet just as I had seen Him work during the birth of each of the first three, I knew He would be faithful again.

Join me now for a closer look into the beautiful ways the Lord can and will use a mother's labor and delivery—from beginning to end—to display His faithfulness and give her joy and the peace that passes all understanding.

Putting Aside the Fear

There are so many horror stories about labor. Pregnant mothers hear all the time about the intense pain, the endless waiting, and all the things that could go wrong. So it's no wonder so many first-time moms go into labor extremely fearful. They need other Christian women to come alongside them and encourage them in the opportunities this experience holds to draw the mom closer to the Lord and point others to Him, no matter what happens. That is what I'm hoping to do for you by sharing my own experiences, passing along helpful insights from other women who have also walked through this, and providing you some practical ways to prepare for this beautiful, life-changing, life-giving event.

God desires to use every single experience we walk through in life—good or bad, easy or difficult, filled with happiness or fraught with deep pain—to sanctify His children and make us more like Him. This includes the labor and delivery process. But it has to be a conscious choice on our part to allow Him to work through our life events as He sees fit. It doesn't just happen.

During the early months of my first pregnancy, I spent many quiet hours on my own, pondering what was to come. I constantly dwelt on that day in June when we would be meeting our first child. There were so many questions and wonderings about the unknown. Would I be able to handle the pain? What if there were a problem? Call us crazy, but we were going to leave the plush, comfortable hospitals of the West to have the birth in Southeast Asia, where my family lives. Yes, this did get a lot of funny reactions from our friends and neighbors. But because my mom had given birth to two children there, we knew the medical care was good. However, there would still be hurdles to clear such as language barriers and vastly different administrative procedures.

God laid it on our hearts when our little one was just the size of a plum to begin praying for the entire labor and delivery process. He began giving us a vision for how He could use this birth to point the doctors, nurses, and hospital staff to Him. So Judah and I began committing this to the Lord in prayer together. As we did, an amazing thing began happening inside me. Rather than growing more and more anxious or fearful as the day drew closer, I was actually excited about what was coming. Because we had been so intentional about looking forward to what the Lord would do, *that* is what I often found myself dwelling on instead of all the unknowns I was facing.

It's amazing what happens when we choose to focus on the eternal rather than fretting over the what-ifs of a situation. As humans, it's not unnatural for us to stew over a major challenge, obstacle, or test that stands before us and dwell on the pain or hardship we might experience as a result. We can easily frighten ourselves to the point that we exclude any expectation of a joyful outcome; we just want to "make it through." On our own in that moment, if we insist on doing what's natural from a human perspective, we have no power to see beyond the potential for pain to grasp or even consider what wonderful thing God may be planning to accomplish through this trial.

It's no different with birthing a baby. Yes, childbirth can be very painful. Yes, it can take hours or even days to bring that baby into the world. Yes, it often means days or weeks of sleepless nights as contractions continually jar us awake and our backs ache because our bellies are almost too big for us to roll from one side to the other. Yes, we might experience some unexpected complication or extended recovery. And yes, something might happen to the baby that we never anticipated. But if we choose to dwell on these things, the anxiety can be paralyzing. Meanwhile, we completely lose sight of the beautiful, joyful miracle that's about to happen! Why then insist on shifting trust away from our all-powerful, all-knowing, never-changing God and placing it instead on vapors? If we will choose to look at the ordeal from an eternal perspective and place our worries into the loving hands of our Lord and then stand back and watch Him work, it changes everything.

My prayer is that you will take away from these pages a vision for the beauty of childbirth and how God wants to use your labor and upcoming delivery. I'm going to share with you some thoughts and practical tips that I hope will be of help to you, but ultimately, I long for you to use this chapter to turn to the Lord in greater dependence than ever before. I know that in Him you will find an unshakeable strength and depth to His love that you can never reach the end of. I pray that by the time of your blessed event, you will have come to know, more than ever before, His love and care for you, His cherished daughter.

Spiritual Birth Likened to Physical Birth

It should come as no surprise that God designed the entire procreation process, from conception to gestation to the act of bringing children into the world. This knowledge should bring you much peace of mind before, during, and after labor, simply knowing that He is in complete control.

Scripture contains many correlations between physical birth and spiritual life. For example, Jesus speaks to Nicodemus of being "born again" in John 3:3–8. And there are many references in the Old Testament in which inner turmoil is likened to being in labor. Isaiah 42:14 provides us an incredible example of God feeling this turmoil as He looks upon the sin of His people: "For a long time I have held my peace; I have kept still and restrained myself; now I will cry out like a woman in labor." This leads first to His wrath being poured out in verse 15, but then we are privy to His beautiful description of what follows:

> *"And I will lead the blind in a way that they do not know, in paths that they have not known I will guide them. I will turn the darkness before them into light, the rough places into level ground. These are the things I do, and I do not forsake them"* (Isaiah 42:16).

Are these verses not a vivid illustration of the turmoil involved in bringing forth a child? There is, arguably, no greater physical pain we will ever experience as women. But the joy that erupts once that process is completed is indescribable! How amazing is it then that this is what spiritual birth is likened to? Is it not often long and painful walking through the steps of surrendering our lives to the Lord? Yet the end result is more beautiful than we can know or even imagine in this lifetime.

Even though the pain of labor is a result of the Fall, when sin entered the world through the disobedience of Adam and Eve (Genesis 3:16), God desires to redeem this pain and use it for His glory—just as He does with every aspect of a Christian's life. It's often in the most difficult of times that His power shines most brightly.

I highly encourage you to look into Scripture and search out the parallels between spiritual and physical birth. If nothing else, you will have a greater understanding of who our God is and just how much we can trust Him and rest in His sovereign plan.

Prayerful Preparation

I cannot overemphasize the importance of fervent prayer as you prepare for your labor and delivery. As new parents go through the usual steps of attending birthing classes, reading books, preparing a birth plan, and assembling the mother's hospital bag, prayer is somehow the one critical component of preparation most needed yet often overlooked.

Any woman who has given birth can attest that there is no way to control every aspect of the process. Even with the smoothest of deliveries, there will almost always be something that doesn't go as planned. We have no idea how long our labor will last, whether the child will be early or late or right on time, whether the nurse we are assigned is attentive or somewhat neglectful, or whether the doctor will arrive on time. Any number of other things could go an unexpected direction. Meanwhile, every emotion, every thought, every choice is intensified during labor, making it difficult to think coherently without becoming anxious or overwhelmed.

That's one of the reasons it's so important to cover the process and participants in prayer during the months leading up to the birth. Prayer operates most powerfully not at those times when we are prepared, but when we are not. When we have been asking the Lord for weeks and months to use this birth for His glory, and to give us His perspective no matter what difficulties arise, then we will be much more likely to hold tight to His hand and trust Him when the unexpected happens.

No issue is too small to bring before the Lord in prayer. If you're not sure whether to choose a hospital or a birthing center, pray and ask the Lord for guidance. If you're feeling overwhelmed by fear, confess that to the Lord and ask Him to fill your heart instead with His peace. If you're concerned that you'll be unable to control your words or actions during the birth, ask God to give you supernatural self-control on that day to only speak and act in a way testifies to His love and life in you. Pray that you and your husband will communicate clearly in the delivery room, and that he will have insight into your needs before you even speak them. Pray for the staff, the nurses, the doctors. Pray about everything.

God loves to hear each and every cry of His children's hearts, no matter how big or seemingly small the issue. Allow your heart to be drawn to Him in a way it never has before as you spend time in His presence preparing for this beautiful event of bringing a new life into the world.

Fear and Labor

It should come as no surprise to us that fear can have a significant effect on a woman's labor. God designed our bodies to react to how we are doing emotionally, and there are few experiences more intense than childbirth.

Most modern childbirth preparation methods have developed from a theory known as the "fear-tension-pain cycle," which says that fear causes tension, and tension increases pain. It's now widely accepted that fear can prolong the childbirth process and actually cause the contractions to be more painful.[1] Not only does fear cause additional physical, mental, and emotional stress, but it can also cause the mother to take her eyes off God.

All of the verses in Scripture concerning fear still apply during labor, perhaps especially so. During labor and delivery, it's very important that we remember God is in control, that He "has not given us a spirit of fear, but of power and of love and of a sound mind" (2 Timothy 1:7, nkjv). This is a truth we can cling to as childbirth intensifies and we are tempted in those moments to wonder how we will get through it.

Fear can be brought on by many things. For first-time moms, it may be the unknowns of the experience combined with any "horror stories" they may have heard. For others, it may be a traumatic experience from a past labor. Still others fear that their child may have a medical condition that results in lifelong complications or even a life that is taken away too soon. These things are very real and are not to be brushed aside or dismissed as petty. Whatever your situation, God so desires that you come to Him with every concern, fear, and anxious thought, because He is ready and able to comfort you and give you peace. He wants you to cast "all your anxieties on him, because he cares for you" (1 Peter 5:7). There is not one thing that is beyond His knowledge or control.

So whatever your fear or concern may be, I urge you to take it to Jesus. As many times as the fear creeps back in, take it to Him again and again. Some fears require our day-by-day, moment-by-moment surrender of things we have difficulty letting go of. Be assured the Lord will be faithful to show you His power and the perfection of His peace in the midst of even the most raging storm.

Here are a few more thoughts on preparing practically to deal with your fear of childbirth:

- Pray. Take each fear, worry, and anxious thought to the Lord. Confess it and ask Him to replace it with His peace, no matter what circumstances you are facing.

- Meditate on Scripture. Look up verses about fear and memorize them. Compile a list to keep with you to read, or have read to you, in labor. If you're feeling creative, print them out with beautiful graphics and surround yourself with them as you go through labor.

- Ask your husband and friends to continually remind you of truth. I know that sometimes, no matter how often I remind myself of a truth, it just doesn't get through to me the way it does when someone else reminds me of the same thing. Asking people to hold you accountable to stay focused on truth is not a sign that you are failing but, rather, that you are wise enough to recognize we all need people in our lives who continually point us to Jesus. This can be a source of incredible strength in times of stress and difficulty.

Waiting Well

You have probably heard that the final weeks of pregnancy feel longer than the rest of it combined. This has certainly been true for me, especially once I reach thirty-eight weeks and know that the baby is fully developed and ready to enter the world. It's the hardest time for me to maintain a content spirit. The daily, well-meaning queries from others contribute to a slightly unnerving feeling that people are putting pressure on you to "get the show on the road" already.

I had very odd labor patterns with my first couple of pregnancies. I would start having contractions every ten minutes or so *weeks* before the baby actually showed up. With my second baby, I went to the hospital, certain I was in early labor. But after a few hours the contractions subsided. I felt so discouraged. I wanted to give in to self-pity, thinking that people maybe thought I was silly for thinking the baby was coming, that my body just wasn't doing what it was supposed to do. Sometimes I would spend all night bouncing on my exercise ball and praying as one after another contraction came and went, knowing I had to get up in the morning and care for a toddler though I barely had enough energy to walk up the stairs.

This pattern continued for three more weeks. Even my doctor couldn't believe I wasn't going into labor. Talk about being tempted to feel justified in my discontent! But I had spent the entire pregnancy asking the Lord to be glorified in and through my every word and attitude and response, no matter what happened, and I chose during those weeks to fight to keep a right attitude. I had to make a daily, moment-by-moment decision to not give into my feelings (and repent when I did). I knew the only way I could keep the right attitude and perspective as I waited was to fully rely on the Holy Spirit, not my feelings, to carry me through to meeting that baby. I knew that how I acted in the weeks leading up to the birth would have a direct effect on how I responded to the labor and delivery.

At the last doctor's appointment before Jenesis came, my doctor opened the door and exclaimed, "You're still smiling! I fully expected you to be more forlorn." The funny thing is, I didn't even consciously realize I was smiling. Had I been depending on my own strength and willpower, I would almost certainly have been sulky and burst into tears the moment the doctor entered the room.

I ended up waiting another four days for my baby to arrive, but those four days were full of further evidences of God's grace. And the delivery day was as calm and peaceful and joyful as we could have asked for. Rather than entering into that time burdened with loads of frustration and discouragement from the weeks of waiting and false starts, our hearts were rejoicing in the fact that we were meeting our daughter that day.

Waiting is rarely our natural choice. In this "free one-day delivery," instant gratification society, we usually want things *now*, not later. Many of us no longer have the patience to stand in long lines or wait in heavy traffic. We get antsy when a website doesn't load in five seconds! And what's our response? To try to do something—*anything*—to fix it, usually crashing the browser in the attempt.

You may have heard it said that we serve a crockpot God in a microwave world. Life tastes better, and is better for us, when we allow God to do things in His perfect timing. He has designed waiting as a way for us to recognize our limitations, to learn that not everything is within our control. And that is a very good thing. Waiting causes us to seek the Lord, to turn to Him when life is slow to fulfill our desires. Turning to God doesn't necessarily make the waiting easy, but it will grow our trust in Him and love for Him as we see more and more of His faithfulness and goodness revealed to us and in us.

When it comes to birthing babies, it takes as long as it takes. So while you're waiting, just as with fear, put together a list of verses that talk about waiting on the Lord. Post them in strategic places around the house where you will see them often. I like to post them by my bathroom mirror, because I spend a fair amount of time there every morning, putting myself together. Here are a few verses to get you started:

May integrity and uprightness preserve me,
for I wait for you. (Psalm 25:21)

Wait for the LORD; be strong, and let your heart
take courage; wait for the LORD! (Psalm 27:14)

"And now, O Lord, for what do I wait?
My hope is in you." (Psalm 39:7)

Who Should Be in the Delivery Room?

The whole labor-and-delivery process is so very personal. So it's understandable that most women opt to have only their husband and sometimes their mom with them in the room. It's certainly not something most people want (or need) to plan a party around. But my mom's story about inviting a neighbor to her delivery has given me a whole new perspective on how the Lord might choose to use it to impact other people's lives.

I started praying early in my first pregnancy about whom the Lord might want to be there, and He placed my sister on my heart. She is seven years younger than me, and when I got married at a young age, it created some emotional distance between us. But once I got pregnant, a door was very clearly opening for us to relate to one another on a deeper level. My sister was so excited about each new thing that was happening to my body. She had once expressed a desire to become a *doula* one day, and as I prayed, this seemed like a perfect opportunity for her to get a glimpse into what that would be like. The Lord really used that time to grow our friendship, and as she has blossomed into a young woman, we have both grown in our love for the Lord and for one another.

For my second delivery, my mom (who attended my first) was not able to be there, so I asked my mother-in-law to stand in for her. My mother-in-law was walking through chemotherapy at the time, and having her there to witness the birth of her granddaughter at the same hospital where we had learned she had cancer was significant for all of us.

I had also asked a friend of mine to attend the birth, but she ended up going out of town before I delivered the baby. So I prayed about who else God might want to be there. Another dear friend came to mind, and she was able to take some pictures for us. It's amazing to see how the Lord used the experience to knit our hearts together. She also has developed a very sweet relationship with Jenesis, our daughter who was born that day.

If you feel a prompting from the Lord to ask someone to be with you for the delivery, even if it's not something you would normally feel comfortable doing, trust that He will use that in very significant ways. Who knows? Along with a physical birth might also come a spiritual birth as well.

This Grace Is for Everyone

Some readers may argue, "You've had such smooth labors and deliveries, so of course you can say these things. It's easier to have a happy disposition when there are no complications and the labor is relatively fast." It is true that there were no unexpected emergencies, but we didn't know that going into the birth. All we could do was trust in the Lord and walk in obedience to Him no matter what the outcome.

When a friend of mine was expecting her first child, she confided in me that she had some fear surrounding labor. She had heard all the stories. But as a believer, she knew that we are called to not worry or fear the unknown. However, she had never heard any examples of labor being a joyous time. I was able to share with her what the Lord had taught me during the preparation for my first child, and just how beautiful His presence was throughout the process. I also recommended a book I had read between babies one and two. *Redeeming Childbirth* by Angie Tolpin is a very helpful resource written from a Christian perspective.

After my friend had her baby, I was anxious to talk with her about her experience. The labor and delivery had been very long and full of unexpected twists. Yet she told me, "It was amazing! God's presence was so real the entire time. We were filled with so much joy and peace in Him the whole time." This was coming from a woman whose delivery was relatively difficult compared to mine, yet she was able to testify of the same divine grace and comfort I had expressed to her.

The same can be true of you, too. Entrust yourself and the birth of your precious baby into the hands of the One who created you both, and I believe you will see incredible fruit as a result!

Gloria Furman has written so poignantly, "We do not 'trust birth' or our bodies; we place our trust in the living God in whose hand is the life of every living thing and the breath of all mankind (Job 12:10). The Lord himself is our refuge (Psalm 18:1–2), not any training, experience, person, book, facility, method, or plan."[2] I encourage you to read her full article, "10 Convictions About Labor and Birth from a Christian Worldview." It's an encouraging and refreshing perspective on how to approach the labor and delivery from a godly perspective.

Being for Each Other, Not Against Each Other

As a newly expectant mom doing research, it doesn't take long to realize that there are a lot of perspectives out there on where and how to deliver babies. And there is so much criticism and pride surrounding these details, even amongst many Christians. Some women stand firmly by delivering a baby in a hospital with an epidural. Others, outside of an emergency, wouldn't dream of anything but a home birth and refuse to use pain medication of any kind. It grieves me to talk to young a mom who feels as if she has somehow failed because she had a caesarean section, usually because of judgmental comments from other women about a C-section being "less than" a natural birth (even if they didn't mean it that way).

In this day of social media, it's so easy for people to state their opinions in a way that disconnects them from the "consequences" of how their words will be taken by someone else. Oh, this should not be so! Yes, it is a good thing to be ready and willing to offer helpful advice. Yes, it's okay to have opinions on whether it's healthier or safer to do something one way over another. But we must remember that, as sisters in Christ, we are to encourage one another and build each other up (1 Thessalonians 5:11). That means when we approach such sensitive subjects as childbirth with one another, we must do so from a place of love and understanding. The wonder of bringing life into this world is not something that should cause division among us; rather, it is something that should cause us to draw closer together, despite our differences. This is an opportunity for women, particularly mothers, to encourage one another, pray for one another, and point one another back to Jesus.

Along similar lines, those of us who have walked through one or more labors need to be very conscious of how we talk about labor with moms who have yet to go through it. I'm not saying we shouldn't share honestly for the sake of not scaring a first-timer. But I am saying we need to be careful to speak in a way that brings life and proclaims the provision and care of our Lord. If you have ever felt compelled to share a graphic, fearful description of your own or someone else's painful experience, you need to ask the Holy Spirit to reveal to you any wrong thinking you've given in to. Are you speaking out of fear? Disappointment? Resentment that your experience or another's didn't go as planned? Whatever the situation, go to the Lord with it. He can redeem even the most harrowing of experiences for His glory and your good.

He wants to use us as an avenue of grace for others who are preparing to walk through the experience for the first time. Even if you feel that you have nothing practical to offer, you can still be used by the Lord to bless that soon-to-be mom. Something as simple as praying with her and for her can encourage her far more than you may ever know. And if there was anything good about a past experience—the way your husband walked through it with you, something that helped you stay calm, items you were glad you packed in your hospital bag—share *those* things!

If you had a good experience, then say so. Even if you tend to be private about your childbirth experience, please don't hesitate to share something that could be a huge blessing to another woman. Be willing to push through the awkwardness for the sake of giving another a hope-filled, Christ-focused perspective going into this very significant time.

If you have ever lost a child in delivery, I am so very sorry. This is certainly not something that is insignificant or that you need to "get over." Your grief is very real, and the process of how the Lord walks a mother through such a loss will be unique to her. I pray that God will be near to you and comfort you in ways you cannot fully fathom. I also pray that the Lord would use you in significant ways to speak into the lives of other mothers who will experience this loss. God knows your pain and has kept all your tears (Psalm 56:8). And He desires to turn even this most tragic and painful of experiences into an eternal weight of glory (2 Corinthians 4:17).

I have heard from other mothers who have lost a child or walked through a near-death labor (whether the life in question was the mother's or child's) that it is very difficult to face another delivery without dread. If this is your story, God has not forgotten you. And your testimony of trusting in Him is that much greater because of what you have gone through.

Some Final, Practical Suggestions

Bring music. Put together a playlist of calming, worshipful music to play in the background during labor. Even if you ultimately choose not to use it, it's a neat process to consider what songs will be most likely to create a peaceful, praise-filled atmosphere. And you certainly don't have to wait for labor to listen to it. Start listening in those times when the waiting feels long, when you're tempted to fear, when you're exhausted and tired of all the aches and pains of those last days of pregnancy. Even if you end up in a situation where you can't use it during the birth or choose not to, you can listen to it afterward as you recover, remembering God's faithfulness in the weeks leading up to that day.

Create special times with your loved ones. Plan to do some special things in the days of waiting for the little one to come. Because two of my pregnancies ended up running late, those days became extra time to spend with family and enjoy some special outings. I played lots of board games with my siblings as I sat on my exercise ball. To get my walking in, I went on an impromptu shopping outing with mother and sister-in-law. I also used this time to slow down and enjoy extra snuggles with my little guy before his sister came to fill my arms. Think of creative things that will set that time apart as being special for all concerned.

Prepare to use your recovery well. Think about ways you can use your recovery time to bond together as a family. It can be too easy to let late-night feedings and exploding diapers get to you and cause stress for the whole family. Remember that recovery is a time when slowing down is a good thing. Use this time to grow in being a team with your husband. If you have more than one child, use all the extra sitting time as an opportunity to give your other children special attention. Don't feel guilty about engaging in a slower pace of life. See it as a gift and thank the Lord for it!

Remember It's a Love Story!

So what happened when I went into labor with my first child in Southeast Asia? Was all the prayer and preparation worth it? Beyond a shadow of a doubt. No, there was no significant transformation (at least that we could see) in the lives of the nurses or doctors. We didn't really know what they were thinking, as the majority of them could only speak a few words of English. But we do know that Christ was honored by the way we walked through that delivery. From the moment my labor started at 11 p.m. on June 3, I was filled with joy. Almost giddy! I could sense God's presence, and He reminded me with each contraction that this was good. Even as I went into transition, when I began to feel that I couldn't go on any longer, the Lord was right there, reminding me through Judah and my mom that He had brought me this far, and it would soon be over. He encouraged me to keep going and finish well.

And that moment when my little boy was placed in my arms will be forever etched in my memory: the feeling of his tiny, wet, body pressed against me and the joy that flooded my being. And knowing that I had depended upon the Lord and walked in a way that glorified Him made that moment all the sweeter.

As you prepare to give birth, give this very precious, personal, and beautiful event to the Lord. Entrust it to Him, and He will use it for His glory and your good. Those around you will stand back and watch God's faithfulness unfolding right before their eyes. When they see a woman walking through labor with joy and peace, it really will surpass their understanding—and yours, too. He created this life and has known from before time exactly how your birth story was going to play out. Imagine how He will use it to draw others to Him!

Testimony of a Trusting Mama

MICHELLE
Mother of Three

In 2015, my husband and I received the exciting news that we were expecting our first child. As I processed the news, I found myself shocked, thrilled, joyful, and terrified—all in about five minutes! What filled my heart with fear (in a moment when you would expect only rejoicing) was the thought that in less than nine months, I would have to go through labor and give birth to meet this precious baby. Within moments, every horror story I'd ever heard about the pain of labor came rushing back. So my husband and I prayed together, thanking God and asking for peace, and that is where I began my journey to surrender my pregnancy and birth story to the Lord.

Over the next few months, I felt in my heart a growing conviction to give birth to my daughter without medication or unnecessary interventions, yet I was terrified to actually walk that out. This was my first pregnancy, so how I could possibly be qualified to make a decision about what I could handle in a situation I had never experienced?

But God graciously began to reveal to me that it wasn't about what I could handle physically or what I thought I was capable of. It was about trusting Him. He would be with me through every step of labor and delivery. He would give me the endurance, strength, peace, and even joy throughout a physically, mentally, and emotionally challenging time. This was an opportunity to be utterly dependent on Him. Of course, I was soberly aware that just because God was with me and caring for me did not mean I would have a problem-free pregnancy or labor. Yet I was amazed at the peace He gave me even as I processed all of this.

If you find that you're apprehensive as your due date (and labor) approaches, let me share with you what greatly encouraged me in that situation. First of all, I prayed throughout my pregnancy. Any time I felt doubt or worry creeping into my mind, I prayed and held on to this scripture:

Do not be anxious about anything, but
in everything by prayer and supplication
with thanksgiving let your requests be
made known to God. And the peace of
God, which surpasses all understanding,
will guard your hearts and your minds
in Christ Jesus. (Philippians 4:6–7)

Once labor hit, praying throughout my contractions proved invaluable. I felt the Lord's peace so strongly, and I knew my mind was safeguarded the entire time.

Second, I had written out several different scripture verses on cards so that my husband could read them to me during labor. It was so calming and encouraging to hear God's truth spoken in that place—to be reminded again and again of His presence with me—that I found I was even **thankful** for the pain, because every contraction meant we were that much closer to meeting our precious baby girl.

Finally, throughout my pregnancy my husband and I gathered worship songs that reminded us of

God's truth through their lyrics. We brought our playlist with us to the hospital and listened to it as I labored. This helped take my mind off myself and pointed me instead to our gracious and loving God. Even though my labor lasted thirty-nine hours, I was at peace, for the Lord was faithful.

Five short months after our first child was born, we learned we were pregnant again. Even after seeing God's faithfulness in mighty ways during my first pregnancy and delivery, I admit that I found myself fearful again. I'm not proud of it, but seriously wondered, *Was it a fluke? Now that I know what labor is like, can I really do this again?*

God graciously reminded me of many of the same truths He taught me the first time around, and although the circumstances were different with my second daughter, He again gave me the peace that surpasses all understanding.

I can honestly say that the births of my children have been among the most intimate times I've ever experienced with the Lord, and I'm so truly grateful for that. I pray that regardless of how your birth story unfolds, you too would surrender all fear, allow His nearness to be your good, and experience the beautiful intimacy of dependence on your great and glorious God.

BONUS CHAPTERS

The LORD is near to the brokenhearted
and saves the crushed in spirit.
Psalm 34:18

The following chapters address topics I have very little or no experience in, but after prayerful consideration, I feel these are important to include in a book about faith and pregnancy. For each of these chapters, I have asked someone who has been an example to others in this area to write it instead.

These chapters are for women who have walked through infertility or the loss of a child. If this is you, know that I have wept tears for you and grieve deeply over your pain. More importantly, know the Lord is holding you in His hands. As you continue to look to Him, casting yourself upon Him and entrusting every burden to Him, He will bring you great and lasting comfort that is beyond your understanding. He will take what was meant for evil and turn it to good.

If you are a friend to someone who has experienced loss or infertility, be assured that you are a blessing and that your prayers on behalf of your friend are heard. I hope you will find encouragement in these pages.

If you have not walked through the pain of loss or infertility, I pray that you will find here greater understanding and a willingness to love and support those who have.

Heather

11

Shattered Life, Faithful Jesus

Walking Through Loss

by Ervina Yoder

*"The Lord is near to the brokenhearted
and saves the crushed in spirit."*
Psalm 34:18

My labor began late in the evening on the first day of spring. Nine long months of pregnancy, many of them spent bedridden with debilitating morning sickness, had given way to the countdown we'd been waiting for. We were pretty certain this was the day, as I was already a week overdue.

We had bathed this pregnancy and this baby in prayer from the beginning. We had chosen Psalm 91 as our firstborn's special passage of Scripture, and we read it aloud each night before we fell asleep. Waiting until birth to find out the baby's gender was a firm rule; my husband, Kenny, wanted maximum surprise, and eventually, I was won over completely. We had installed a shiplap wall in the neutral-colors nursery, where cozy newborn clothes were hung on the world's tiniest hangers and soft blankets were washed and waiting. We were the world's most excited parents, and our families shared our excitement.

After I lay awake all night with contractions, the sun finally rose on Friday, March 21. We put the finishing touches on our hospital bags, took a long walk to help the process along, and then headed for our midwife's office. I was breathing through waves of pain and desperately hoping I'd have progressed far enough to be admitted to the hospital. I waited in our car to huff and puff in privacy while Kenny checked at the receptionist desk to see if we could bypass the normal wait and be seen immediately. Successful in his quest, he came back for me, and we headed to a back room where the doctor engaged in cheerful conversation as she applied jelly to the Doppler and swiped it over my stomach, waiting for the familiar *swoosh, swoosh, swoosh* of a heartbeat. After a long moment of silence, she switched the instrument from one side to the other, then down to the bottom, then up to the top. My heartrate spiked with a jolt of fear I refused to entertain even as we were whisked to another room with ultrasound equipment.

My contractions were five minutes apart when we found out our baby no longer had a heartbeat.

In a moment—in the two seconds it took for the doctor to say the words—the air was sucked from the room. Time stood still as our joy turned to stunned panic. Where there should have been a stretching, kicking child eager to exit his home of nine months, the ultrasound screen showed only a lifeless form. The doctor left the room to give us privacy. My contractions intensified as Kenny stretched his shaking hands over my stomach and whispered sobbing prayers. "Please, please restore life. . . ."

I gave birth that day, and the next I watched my husband shovel dirt onto a tiny grave. I had gone from the heights of expectancy to the depths of shock, grief, and the unimaginable pain of never seeing my firstborn son take a breath. I cannot describe the agony of sorrow, but I can describe God's faithfulness in the midst of it.

From the moment the ultrasound confirmed our worst fear and the doctor's words, "Your baby's not alive," a grace and peace were poured into Kenny and me that is unexplainable apart from Jesus Christ.

Comfort in Community

Hours after Little Kenny was born, our families had arrived from five different states to hold him and hold us. My dad made dozens of calls and took care of funeral arrangements, asking us only necessary questions but removing the burden of making hard decisions. When we dreaded going home to an empty house, Kenny's parents had already decided to spend the next few nights and take care of any little thing we needed. Friends showed up at our door, understanding if we needed space but letting us know they weren't afraid of being with us in our grief. We were covered in prayer, surrounded in friendship, and showered with meals. Our mailbox overflowed with handwritten letters for weeks, and within a few days a weeklong trip for Kenny and me was fully funded through the kindness of friends and strangers. Do not underestimate the impact that the body of Christ can have on hurting souls. It is a very real and beautiful thing.

Comfort in Scripture

I've heard a vast array of opinions on grieving—mamas who speak of their losses and the ways they've been affected, the ways they've coped, the ways they've healed. I came across a blog written by a popular Christian speaker and songwriter, who had also tragically lost a baby. She wrote about she disliked that many people "beat themselves over the head with Bible verses" when they were grieving instead of "just being real" about how hard it was. She recounted how she would often lose herself in entertainment, relieved she didn't have to face her painful reality while binge-watching seasons of mindless shows. Reading her perspective, I felt so much sadness. In the flesh, it makes sense, because the desire can be strong to retreat into mind-numbing activities. But what about afterward? Where is the refreshment of soul for one who has sought refuge in the things of the world instead of the things of Jesus? Where is the measure of healing after the short-lived coping mechanism is gone and the weight of sorrow slams you again?

When Christ faced His darkest hour, where did He turn? To prayer. To His Father. He begged for the cup to be removed, yes, but He nonetheless submitted and chose to walk the path that lay ahead, entrusting Himself to the care and purposes of God. For me, Scripture was not a spiritual baseball bat I used to intensify my pain or a pious Band-Aid to cover my raw and open wound; instead, the Word became my lifeline. For months, there were many days when I could only read the Psalms, but they spoke for my heart when I came before the Lord in weeping agony.

I feel strongly that, contrary to what our culture proclaims, authenticity doesn't have to mean negativity. It is possible to be honest and genuine about the reality of your heartache while claiming the healing comfort and sweet companionship that comes from being deeply rooted in Jesus and His Word. It's not in the job description of a secular world to provide long-lasting comfort, stability, and hope when the hurt is beyond our control, but it is the very nature of Jesus.

Comfort in a Firm Foundation

I never wanted to be a woman who understands heartbreak at a deep and personal level. I never wanted to be acquainted with the intense sadness of not getting to know my child on earth. But there is no greater richness than to have life fall apart and still be unshaken because of the foundation of knowing who God is. Having His truth and His promises sustain me gave me an assurance of His presence that I'd never felt before. In the agonizing grief of giving our baby back to Jesus, I leaned the weight of my grief on the steady shoulders of Jesus and found Him to be so near, so faithful, so sufficient, so redeeming.

Psalm 18:30 (NKJV) says, "As for God, His way is perfect." Do I believe that, with a full-term pregnancy and a labor that turned into my worst nightmare? Do I believe there are no mistakes, no accidents, nothing outside of His control? I don't believe the Lord took our son's life; that is against His very nature and character. But I do believe He allowed our child to be taken for reasons not yet known (and never fully known on this earth), except that He will work this loss for our good and for His glory. I believe that because I couldn't have survived such pain if I didn't. Because this is who I know Him to be. Because He is the hope that anchors my soul. Because the way before me is not untrodden: Jesus was "a man of sorrows and acquainted with grief." Surely He has borne my griefs and carried my sorrows (Isaiah 53:3–4). If He took on the weight of sin and endured the cross so grace would triumph, if God could turn the anguish of the cross into love's greatest accomplishment, how much more can He use any moment in our lives for His glory and the good of His children? As Charles Spurgeon wrote, "And so, believing that God rules all, that he governs wisely, that He brings good out of evil, the believer's heart is assured, and he is enabled calmly to meet each trial as it comes."[1]

We cannot look to ourselves to find what we need to withstand the worst of life. We simply do not have what it takes. Following Little Kenny's death, well-meaning people would hug me and say, "You're so brave" or "You're so strong." These were meant as compliments, yet I was anything but. I was tremendously fragile and weak in my heartache.

If You're Caring for a Friend

Grief is raw and unpredictable, and it can feel awkward to enter into someone else's loss. If you have a friend who is grieving the loss of her baby, be sensitive to her loss, but please don't feel like you need to tiptoe around your grieving friend.

Pray with and for her often, but also love her in practical ways. Listen to the promptings of the Holy Spirit and act on them, whether it's sending a simple text saying you're remembering her and her baby today, offering to do her grocery shopping, dropping off a meal, picking up her kids for the day, giving her flowers, writing a note, or sharing a scripture. Let her know you're available to come take a walk or bring coffee. Invite her family over for supper, but understand if they need their space. Talk with her about her baby. Ask how she's doing and be ready to listen. These are gestures of comfort and sweetness and blessing. Don't feel like you need to know the right thing to say. What blessed me most in my grief was knowing I was not alone but was surrounded by a community of friends who were not afraid of our pain.

At least a half dozen close friends were due within a month of my giving birth, and I knew I had a choice: I could stay away and isolate myself from their joy because it would make me more acutely aware of what was missing from my life, or I could be intentional about coming alongside my friends and rejoicing with them. I'm thankful these sweet friends didn't hold me at arm's length but readily extended invitations to spend time with their families. It was healing to walk into their hospital rooms and homes and embrace their newborn bundles, tears of sorrow mingling with tears of awe and wonder at the sheer miracle of life. So often, celebration and sorrow seem to go hand in hand, and it is only by the wisdom and grace of our Lord that we learn to balance them well.

Comfort at Home

After my baby died, I questioned my very identity. I was a mother, yet not a mother. Mine was a body filled, then emptied. There were times I would venture out to buy groceries or walk through Target and realize that no one there knew I was a mom. I wanted to wear a shirt or a banner, something that testified I had given birth and there should be an adorable baby in my cart!

It was a crushing, aching loneliness, and I had very real, very honest questions: *Where do I go from there? What does my life even mean anymore? Who am I without my long-anticipated child?* Meanwhile, my husband was struggling with questions of his own.

Most of us have heard stories or known of heartbreaking situations in which marriages were torn asunder by the death of a family member. This kind of loss takes parents to a place of profound emotional pain and spiritual wrestling, and this was true of Kenny and me. However, by God's grace, our grief also drove us to a place of deeper unity as husband and wife. When emotions are raw in the wake of tragedy, even the smallest misunderstanding or frustration can easily lead to hurt and the building of walls, but our closeness was the work of God. It was a sweet gift we did not take for granted.

I would caution you as a wife to be careful not to place unrealistic expectations on your husband in the midst of devastating loss. Praise God if he is a man who leads you tenderly and faithfully through the maze of heartache and emotions, but he cannot be all things for you. He was never meant to be. My husband was a strong and steady support, but even so, there were days when his grieving looked quite different from mine, and I had to lay down my expectations of how I wanted to be cared for, or what I was wanting him to be feeling and expressing, or the ways I was hoping to commemorate our baby's birthday.

New Chances to Trust

Four years later, we have been given two more precious children, Harrison Jude and Eleanor Kate—daily reminders of God's goodness and two more opportunities to trust in His wisdom and care. Each pregnancy was a constant battle against fear, and it took focused, continual discipline for me to take such thoughts captive and remind myself of truth. Often I would wake in the middle of the night, wait for a kick or stirring, feel nothing, then start to succumb to the paralyzing grip of fear. I would wake Kenny and ask him to pray for the baby and me. He so kindly (and groggily) would, and then I could go back to sleep in peace.

Because we were never given clear answers for Little Kenny's death, there was no sigh of relief after arriving at a certain milestone, no "safe" trimester. Each day was a gift to be treasured. Yes, I monitored fetal movement more closely during these pregnancies, and our care providers urged us to come in for frequent ultrasounds. But I quickly realized that I had no more control over these pregnancies than I had with our first. So although I did my best to steward and nurture the developing life I was carrying, I learned to recognize morning sickness, the physical discomfort, and the painful labor and delivery for what they were: reminders to surrender my full confidence to the Lord who knows the measure of my days and those of my children.

Now my days are filled with child training and oatmeal baking, chin wiping and floor cleaning, cheek kissing and story reading. Kenny and I remember and miss our firstborn son fiercely, but with his memory we call to mind the restoration that has been woven through our story ever since. God truly redeems those whose desire it is to serve and honor Him. He gives me everything I need to walk through the valley of death, fearing no evil, for He is with me.

Today heaven seems closer, and I'm realizing just how much of a shadow this life is compared to the glorious reality of eternity.

The truth is, motherhood is not my life. Jesus is my life. And because He lives, for me to live is Christ. He is stripping me of my comfort and pleasure in this world and giving me a longing for the one to come. Until His return, you and I must be intentional about steadying our hearts in a fallen world, searching the Scriptures daily to know more firmly the character and person of our God. We must build our faith on a foundation of truth instead of allowing emotions and circumstances to dictate and dominate our theology. We must carry our burdens to Him and allow our broken, humble lives to witness to the world how good and faithful our trustworthy God is.

12

Healing a Barren Heart

Walking Through Infertility

by Jasmin Howell

"I have heard your prayer; I have seen your
tears. Behold, I will heal you."
2 Kings 20:5

God alone knows why we never conceived. Yes, we underwent some testing, only to be told that, physiologically, we were totally normal. Our infertility journey did not involve a plethora of tests, in-vitro attempts, or intensive hormone therapies. That may be your story, however, and that's okay. My infertility journey is one of many and has its own plot twists, experiences, and emotional highs and lows. In God's masterful design, no two stories are alike among His children.

I was reminded of this truth recently while having coffee with a friend who struggled with infertility for ten years before eventually carrying her in-vitro baby girl to term, whereas my journey with infertility ended in an adoption. Our stories may be different, but I believe that every woman who struggles with infertility shares a common thread—the grief and loss we feel and the fact that we must eventually reckon it with the gospel of Christ.

That's the part of my story I want to share.

The Seed—Fall 2014

After arriving late to church that memorable Sunday, my husband, Mike, and I settled into a pew just as the pastor was inviting a number of women to the stage. "We want to pray over these women," he said, as they arranged themselves in a line, "and praise God for the joy of new life. Each of these precious women is expecting a baby in the next few months!"

Of course I knew that a few women in our congregation were expecting, but Mike and I had been away at Bible school that summer, and the significance of the announcement didn't fully hit me until I saw these five women standing together, round bellies side by side. The pastor continued, "Even as we praise God for these gifts, we want to remember those in our congregation who desire children yet remain childless." As he started to pray for the women on stage, instead of closing my eyes, I glanced around at our small congregation. I felt like someone had just turned a white-hot spotlight on me. *He's talking about us*, I thought. *We are the only childless ones left.*

It was true, at least in part. Mike and I had been married for seven years but had not been successful in conceiving. Now, with the birth of these five babies, my husband and I would be the only young couple in our church who did not have children. Most of my friends were already working on their second, third, or fourth babies, yet my womb and arms remained empty. The march of time had not escaped my notice as I crossed over into my thirties.

I summoned the willpower to stay in the pew, as slipping out might reveal the true depth of pain that the pastor's prayer had touched in me. Hot tears took me by surprise, and I wiped them away before they could be noticed. Even though every head was bowed in prayer, I felt as though they were all watching me, the barren one.

That's when I felt a whispered accusation from the enemy: *God must not love you to keep this blessing from you.*

I wish I could say I immediately identified it as a lie, or that I rejected it at once. But I did neither. I had struggled awhile with this issue of infertility, and I was growing more and more concerned, especially as people seemed to be asking more and more frequently when we were planning to have children.

The months that followed that Sunday service were among the most difficult of my adult life. A little seed had been planted in my heart that day that pointed to my infertility as evidence that I was unloved, unworthy, rejected, and alone. The seed grew another little root every time I dwelled upon this thought.

And the baby announcements just kept coming. In addition to the five women at church, three more friends shared the news that they were expecting their first babies. These followed on the heels of both of my younger sisters giving birth for the first time. My lack of a child could not have been made more glaring. After seven years of marriage, I was feeling pretty far behind my peers in terms of starting a family.

One of the biggest lies I faced was feeling that I had "failed" at the next step of my life. Once a woman is married, it seems as if everybody wants to know, "When are you having kids?" It's a normal expectation but a hard one to bear when "normal" doesn't happen. And the more time passes, the more abnormal a woman feels.

I was struggling with being the childless one in the midst of so many new mothers, but I was careful to keep my feelings hidden, because I didn't want to burden anyone with my grief or draw further attention to my failure. I already resented how my husband and I stuck out like a sore thumb in our community. As the object of many people's sympathy, prayers, and concern, I didn't want any of it. I just wanted a baby, like everyone else had.

The Roots

All my life I had believed that God was good, and my life experiences up to that point had seemed to confirm my belief. Mine had been a life of relative ease and happiness. In that context, it was easy to believe God's Word and trust Him. Now, however, my faith was being put to the test. Suddenly, I found that all my belief and trust hinged on one question that I kept asking over and over: *Is He good to me?* Could I still believe He loved me when He seemed to be callously withholding the single greatest desire of my heart, while forcing me to watch as He generously poured out abundant blessings on the women around me? This seemed unbearably cruel.

I began wallowing in hopelessness and indulging in self-pity, while finding it harder and harder to pray. Meanwhile, my Bible lay unopened.

I honestly tried to rejoice with those who were rejoicing, though I was mourning inside, but pain battered my heart with every baby shower I attended and every piece of conception advice I received from a well-meaning friend ("Have you tried such-and-such?"). I was feeling unloved and unchosen, and my empty womb was my evidence. The roots of these thoughts continued to grow in strength until I could no longer remember what the seed had been.

The temptation was intense to completely withdraw—from God, my church, my husband, my friends and family. I began closing myself off from the Lord's comfort and letting my grief swallow me instead. My heart, previously so tender and responsive to the working of the Lord, now grew cold and hard as I kept asking, *Is He good to me?* To my eyes, all the evidence seemed to say no.

I didn't even realize I was asking the wrong question.

When I did manage to open my Bible, I kept stumbling across verses about the blessings of motherhood, birth, and family. These only discouraged me further, none more so than Psalm 127:3, "Behold, children are a heritage from the LORD, the fruit of the womb a reward." Through the broken lens of my hurt and anger, the implications of this verse seemed so harsh: The Lord gave children to those He wanted to reward, to those who were deserving, but somehow, my husband and I had been … what, disqualified?

Now, not only was I grieving, but I was angry. The darkness I was descending into scared me, but I had no idea what to do about it. Those roots had their tendrils wrapped around my heart, and I couldn't disentangle myself.

The Uprooting—Winter 2014

I am so thankful for the Lord's grace and mercy. Despite my unrighteous, self-centered anger, He was working to gently draw me back to Himself. And in a single moment, one very early morning in December of that year, my heart began to melt.

The night before had been one of the worst of my life. I had been up late and, in a scene reminiscent of Genesis 30:1–2, was furiously venting to my husband in much the same way Rachel exploded at her husband Jacob, saying "Give me children, or I shall die!" Like a too-full pot boiling over, my anger suddenly overflowed in a scalding torrent. I spewed out terrible things that night. Afterward, I cried myself to sleep, feeling utterly hopeless and lost. My husband was at a loss too. He grieved for me and prayed for me but knew he could not fix this.

The next morning, in the very early hours, I climbed out of bed and padded to the dark living room, watching as the gas fireplace flickered in the darkness like the tiny spark of faith still burning in me. The anger of the night before had turned to shame and sorrow. I didn't want to be like this. I desperately wanted to be free from the oppression I felt in my spirit, but I didn't know how.

In Romans 8:26, the apostle Paul explains how the Holy Spirit "helps us in our weakness." When we don't know what to pray for, "the Spirit himself intercedes for us with groanings too deep for words." My spirit burdened and weary, I had truly had come to the end of myself. I certainly did not know how to pray or what to ask for, but in my weakness and uncertainty, I opened my Bible for the first time in months to Proverbs and began reading in chapter 30, as it was the thirtieth day of the month. I can see clearly now how the Spirit guided me to this chapter, both for my freedom and His glory.

My eyes settled on two verses that changed my life drastically:

> *There are three things that are never satisfied, four never say, "Enough!": the grave,* the barren womb, *the earth that is not satisfied with water—and the fire never says, "Enough!"* (Proverbs 30:15–16, NKJV, emphasis mine).

This passage speaks of four things that can never be filled: Hades, or the world of the dead; the barren womb, which cannot host life; the parched desert, whose thirst can never be quenched; and the rampant fire, which consumes everything in its path, always hungry for more. The Hebrew word translated here as *barren* is synonymous with prison restraints and oppression.[1]

I had been feeling so unloved and lonely, so captivated by the lie that I was rejected, an outcast whose prayers went unheard. But as I read this verse, I had instant understanding as only God can give, and I saw the significance of the verse, as though a veil had been lifted from my eyes.

The phrase "the barren womb" seemed to leap off the page, just as I also saw that it was surrounded by three other concepts: hell, a desert, and a consuming fire. As I read the passage again, the Lord helped me see so clearly: The yawning pit of my empty womb could rob me of abundant life, put me in chains, burn up my joy, and give the devil a foothold in my life—if I let it.

Oh, the great love of the Lord! In His lovingkindness, He brought me to this verse to pierce the darkness with the light of truth and turn my feet to another path. I now saw the seed of the lie that had been planted months ago—that I was unloved and rejected—and how I had allowed it to grow into my sinful anger. And in a moment of great compassion, God snatched up the lie by the roots and threw it into the flames of hell where it belonged. Undeniable truth filled its place: I was *so deeply* loved, with the kind of love a parent shows when he urgently warns his child not to put her hand into a fire. Coming across that verse wasn't a cozy hug, and it didn't give me warm fuzzies. It startled me and grabbed my attention with the seriousness of its consequences. It sharply changed my focus and led me to safety.

I wept as I have never wept! Then I dried my eyes and confessed the anger, frustration, and drowning sorrow of the past months and asked my Savior for His help to be free. I then asked my husband's forgiveness for taking so much of my pain out on him instead of acknowledging its deeper roots. And in both relationships, I received loving forgiveness.

And you know what? My anger left, along with the lie. The tangible presence of the Holy Spirit and the comfort of the Word were a healing balm. My once-barren heart began to grow new life, as the Lord planted seeds of truth in place of the lies I had entertained. He showed me that even what seems like a barren place still holds great potential for beauty in His hands:

> *The wilderness and the dry land shall be glad;*
> *the desert shall rejoice and blossom like the cro-*
> *cus; it shall blossom abundantly and rejoice*
> *with joy and singing. (Isaiah 35:1-2)*

Now I knew with certainty that I was not alone, that the Lord wanted to use my journey of infertility for a purpose, and that He had a plan to give hope and bring forth beauty even within these present hardships. He would not harm me through these circumstances but was with me in them, though He had not removed me from them for purposes far beyond my comprehension (Jeremiah 29:11).

How to Deal with Infertility in Light of the Gospel

As the months passed, I grew content with His plans for me. Slowly, I became aware that *He*—not a baby in my arms—was my reward, my hope, and my peace. If I couldn't be satisfied in Him, I would never be satisfied, no matter the circumstances. So I continually asked to be satisfied.

And the Lord showed me how to deal with my loss in light of the gospel. First I had to grieve it, then surrender it, and then share it with my community.

1. Grieve It

For me, the first step to being satisfied in Christ was to properly recognize and grieve the loss I was facing. I needed to acknowledge the reality that I was not pregnant, that I might never become a mother, and that this was the story God was writing for my life. I also had to accept that, although I might never be a mom, God is still good and His plans are perfect. But grieving was the first step to accepting this, because grieving took me to the foot of the cross.

One day at a time, the Lord began to teach me how to grieve rightly—not apart from Him as I had been doing, but so near to Him that my falling tears wet His feet, as in Luke 7:38. And I wept a *lot*. I wept privately before the Lord, in the arms of my husband, and on the shoulders of my closest friends. As my Savior is acquainted with sorrows and was familiar with mine, taking them to Him became a very real part of worship for me. Not only was I learning where to take my sadness, but I was also learning so much about His character and His comfort through this process. As He unraveled the lies in my life, I was driven to His Word for reassurance of who He was and who I was in Him.

Slowly, I realized an important truth: My sadness and grief were not sins, but how I chose to deal with them had led me into sin. Apart from Christ, these emotions could lead to suffering, damaged relationships, isolation, and anger. But in His company, they could lead me to immeasurable, overflowing life even in the midst of great pain and loss.

I recognized that the only way to be truly free was to take my grief and the feelings of sadness, pain, and emptiness to the Lord and give them to Him as an offering. So when I felt sad, I didn't avoid it. Rather, I invited the Lord to be with me and comfort me. When I felt that pang of deep loss, I didn't hide my face; I turned my face toward Him. When I felt overwhelmed with sorrow, I remembered that His Spirit was praying and interceding for me, and I rested. When I felt tempted to withdraw, I drew near instead.

Verses like this one became frequent, comforting reminders of where my focus should be:

> *Though the fig tree should not blossom, nor fruit be on the vines, the produce of the olive fail and the fields yield no food, the flock be cut off from the fold and there be no herd in the stalls, yet I will rejoice in the LORD; I will take joy in the God of my salvation. (Habakkuk 3:17–18)*

Loss will be part of life in this broken world, and yet I found I had every reason to rejoice because the Lord had poured out His life for me.

2. Surrender It

I daily had to lay down my desire to understand why. Why us? Why didn't we have children? Why did I have to walk through this? Why, why, why? These unanswerable questions had to be laid on the altar. I knew that the next step was to stop wrestling with my reality, lay down my expectations, and embrace what God had given me. This step was much harder because it required the intentional act of taking every thought captive (2 Corinthians 10:5) and choosing to change my focus from what I lacked to what I had in Him.

Previously I had been asking, "Is He good to me?" Now I went to God's Word asking simply, "Is He good?" Adding the qualifier "to me" had caused a downward spiral in my heart because I was focusing on my perception of His goodness only in terms of my desires and the fulfillment of them. I had been seeking evidence of God's goodness only in my experiences and not in His Word.

Removing "me" from the equation allowed me to surrender my experiences and stop wrestling with them. This change in perspective wondrously opened up the Word for me in a whole new way, revealing that the absolute goodness, righteousness, and justness of God were indivisible from His very nature. When I started to see Him properly through His word, I also began to see how He was working, present, and faithful in my experiences.

3. Share It

The most difficult seasons of our lives, even those filled with often unbearable pain, have the potential to be useful in the kingdom of God. He desires always to grow us in love and knowledge of Himself and to use our lives to reveal deep and profound truths about His nature. But it is wiser to acknowledge our difficulties and share them with others than to struggle privately and alone. We should feel the pain as deeply as we must but not hide from those who love us and thereby quench what God may want to use it for in our lives and in the lives of others.

Unless I fled to the wilderness and became a hermit living in a cave, there was just no escaping my community, which was peopled largely by mothers with full arms and those who were pregnant. I was a people person, and these people were my people. I loved them all, and I wanted to rejoice in what God was doing in their lives without hesitation.

I now recognized that I could not walk through this journey of infertility alone. In addition to confiding in my husband, I began to show up and share my heart with my community of other women. I asked them for prayer in this area of hurt and shared the deepest burdens of my heart with women I knew would listen, comfort, encourage me in truth, and sometimes just cry with me. My husband and I also had a few meetings with our church leaders to share with them. The knowledge that we were surrounded by prayer was so comforting!

In community, there is not only comfort but also the relief of unburdening our hearts, the beauty of fellowship, and being rejuvenated together in the Spirit. We may have all been at different stages of life, but the friendships I enjoyed with the women in my life were strong because of our differences. Our common foundation was faith in Jesus, and that was more than enough to bless us mightily.

For months, I had viewed my struggles as being *extra* difficult. Bringing my needs to my community brought light to the pain that others were facing for different, though no less difficult, reasons. Being in community opened my eyes to the needs of those around me, to their joys and sorrows, and gave me a reason to reach out in love beyond my natural capacity, beyond my own hurt. Yes, my journey was unique and precious in God's sight, but my hardships were not "extra special hardships." Being in community reminded me that hardship is as common to the Christian as breathing, and yet within our fellowship is found a sustaining courage that comes not from all our problems being solved, but from turning our eyes collectively to our Savior and drawing strength from His Word and His body of believers.

Looking back, I understand the significance of the Lord's placing me and my empty womb in the midst of so many pregnancies and expanding families. Never can our own emptiness be seen so drastically except when viewed in contrast to fullness. Through immense grief, God was crafting a wonderful testimony of grace in my life, my marriage, and my relationships.

The only way to journey to the other side of a valley is *through*, but we were not meant to walk through the valley alone. By sharing the burden of our sorrows with one another, we can receive the blessing that is the love of a Christian community. Our brothers and sisters may not be able to relate to every tiny detail of our troubles, and they may not perfectly comfort us or provide flawless encouragement. But they will, I believe, lighten our load while pointing us to the truth.

Even if...

I only know one thing for sure about my infertility: It revealed more about my heart than it did about my womb.

The emptiness and the unmet longings I felt eventually led me to an entirely different question: Would I allow the Spirit to fill up what I could not? Would I allow Him to fill me with the very real and overflowing life He offered? *Even if* that life never included my own child? *Even if* our lives looked different from what we considered normal? *Even if* we were the only childless couple in our community? *Even if* this meant relinquishing my own plans and dreams and clinging to Him for His sake alone?

Oh, how I wrestled with this question. I had to reevaluate a lot of things, specifically my relationship with the Lord, errors in my understanding of His Word and His character, and the deeper motivations of my own heart. Was I going to follow the Lord *only* if He gave me what I wanted? Would I trust Him *only* if the result was happiness, not suffering? As I read His word, I discovered the truth that a closed womb, closed for the

Lord's purposes, cannot be opened except by Him. Fertility treatments, health products, family planning methods, medical advances—these cannot open the womb or create a hospitable environment for a pregnancy. *Only* the Lord can do this, though He will lead us in wisdom and may choose to provide through various earthly means.

We must trust first and foremost in the sovereignty of God and not in our own wisdom or the wisdom of the world. And like every other gift that is given to us—or withheld from us—on this earth, we must choose in what or whom we will put our hope and trust. What will we proclaim about the Lord, especially when life doesn't seem to live up to our expectations, plans, and dreams?

I learned more about the care of my heavenly Father in the valley of infertility than I ever did on the more easily traveled paths of my life. The truth is that a barren womb does not have to result in a barren heart. Whether there is never a child, or if a child arrives through medical intervention, through choosing to adopt, or by a natural pregnancy down the road, full joy is absolutely possible! Life flows from a woman who has found her complete satisfaction in the plans of God, who rests in His goodness and trusts in His love for her—even if.

Note from Heather: To their shock and amazement, Jasmin and her husband, Mike, learned in January 2020 that they are expecting a baby after thirteen years of marriage. With God, all things are possible (Matthew 19:26)!

Special Thanks

A special thanks goes to the many people who helped make this book a reality through their generous giving, including Beth Livingstone, Carey Christian, Marissa Price, Haley Parson, Naomi Vacaro, Mickey and Trina Cofer, Caleb and Jeannie Sprenger, Barrie Greenfield, Eric and Kim Stump, Collin and Lynnelle Peters, Katrina Parsons, Jake and Laura Redding, Cameron and Dorian Sprenger, Ben and Rochele Griffin, Bob and Claire Knapp, Jon and Kathy Haley, Mark and May Kramer, Rebecca Spaulding, Holly Sprenger, Caroline Heath, Brandon and Jess White, Andy and Laurel Sprenger, Gloria Boldt, Mike and Carol Beth Sprenger, Rebekah Walton, Karl Kine, Cassidy Shooltz, Darius and Monica Tantanella, Aubry and Jesse Skelton, Shawn and Shelli Kibler, Michaela Gothman, Mike and Jasmin Howell, Dave and Kathy Heggland, Joel and Lydia Duke, Stacy Stutzman, Joann Mullett, Jen Roseman, Timari Deane, Allison Tonkin, Nawon Losli, Les and Eileen Sprenger, Michael and Cristina Morgan, Brandon and Gabrielle Golden, John and Suzanne Dalrymple, Keith and Kim Sprenger, and Rachel Baker.

Notes

Introduction

1 Noah Webster, *An American Dictionary of the English Language* (New York: S. Converse, 1828).

Chapter 1

1 In the years following my diagnosis with Polycystic Ovarian Syndrome, I was told by other doctors that this had been a misdiagnosis. Whether it was a misdiagnosis or the Lord healed my body, I do know that God used that those circumstances to bring me to a place of greater trust in Him.

Chapter 2

1 *Chicago Tribune*, "The health benefits of singing a tune," March 15, 2018.

Chapter 3

1 *This Momentary Marriage: A Parable of Permanence,* John and Noel Piper (Wheaton, IL: Crossway Books, 2009).

Chapter 5

1 Nancy DeMoss Wolgemuth, *My Personal Petitions Prayer Journal* (Niles, MI: Revive Our Hearts, 2016).

Chapter 6

1 "Fetal Alcohol Spectrum Disorders (FASDs): Alcohol Use in Pregnancy," *Centers for Disease Control and Prevention,* www.cdc.gov/ncbddd/fasd/alcohol-use.html.

2 "Caffeine in Pregnancy," *March of Dimes,* www.marchofdimes.org/pregnancy/caffeine-in-pregnancy.aspx.

3 Hannah Whitall Smith, *The God of All Comfort,* Christian Classics Ethereal Library, www.ccel.org/ccel/smith_hw/comfort.html.

Chapter 7

1 Leslie Ludy, "Exchanging Chaos for Strength, Part Three: Letting Motherhood Challenges Make You Strong," *Set Apart Motherhood,* http://setapartmotherhood.com/devotional/christ-centered-mothering/exchanging-chaos-for-strength.

2 Jani Ortlund, *Fearlessly Feminine: Boldly Living God's Plan for Womanhood* (Colorado Springs, CO: Multnomah Books, 2000).

3 Nancy DeMoss Wolgemuth, "Does Physical Beauty Matter?," *Revive Our Hearts,* www.reviveourhearts.com/articles/does-physical-beauty-matter.

Chapter 8

1 Jen Wilkin, "Why Hospitality Beats Entertaining," *The Gospel Coalition,* April 9, 2016, www.thegospelcoalition.org/article/why-hospitality-beats-entertaining.

2 Elisabeth Elliot, *A Lamp unto My Feet* (Ventura, CA: Regal Books, 2004), p. 16.

3 John Piper, "Strategic Hospitality," *Desiring God,* August 25, 1985, www.desiringgod.org/messages/strategic-hospitality.

Chapter 10

1 "What About Pain?," *University of Minnesota,* www.takingcharge.csh.umn.edu/explore-healing-practices/holistic-pregnancy-childbirth/what-about-pain.

2 Gloria Furman, "10 Convictions About Labor and Birth from a Christian Worldview," *The Gospel Coalition,* January 5, 2016, www.thegospelcoalition.org/article/10-convictions-about-labor-and-birth-from-a-christian-worldview.

Chapter 11

1 C. H. Spurgeon, "Morning, August 5," *Morning and Evening* (New Kensington, PA: Whitaker House, 2001).

Chapter 12

1 Strong's Concordance, Hebrew Dictionary, #H6115.

For more from Heather Cofer, visit her website

heathercofer.com